Updated   and   Expanded   Edition

I0104475

Christine Danella Lynch

More Than
Tender Points:
A Fibromyalgia Memoir

**With Discussion Questions
for FM Support Groups**

Medical Disclaimer: Treatments and therapies described in this book may not be appropriate for your unique condition and diagnosis and should in no way replace the services of a qualified health professional. Utilization of any advice taken from this book is entirely at the reader's discretion.

ISBN-13: 978-0-9790534-0-5
ISBN-10: 0-9790534-0-4

Table of Contents

About Support Groups

About Disability

About Life with Fibromyalgia

Appendices

Introduction

So many changes have occurred in the field of fibromyalgia (FM) since Tender Points: A Fibromyalgia Memoir was published in 2007 that even a title change was required to write a second edition. The abbreviation of FMS is also no longer valid since fibromyalgia is no longer considered to be a syndrome (a collection of symptoms). Rather, it is now an entity of its own. Therefore, the correct abbreviation has become FM.

The original Tender Points has been enhanced and updated with current knowledge and experience that I've gained in the past eleven years. More Than Tender Points contains much more information on alternative or "complementary" forms of medicine. Additional topics include acupuncture and acupressure, pain management, nutrition and supplements, medical cannabis, avoiding the "sickness culture", the importance of attitude, and entire chapters on support groups and food. Even the original chapters incorporate new, up-to-date information about FM as well as additional (and quite unusual) experiences I have undergone as a result of having this illness. Basically, it's a whole new book.

An article I was invited to write for Fibromyalgia and Chronic Pain Life Magazine (2011 Nov./Dec. edition) explains in detail the additions to the diagnostic criteria made by the American College of Rheumatology

(ACR) that year and explains why those changes were made. The result is that today, symptoms such as IBS, fatigue, sleep disturbances and cognitive difficulties are also considered in the diagnostic process.

Anyone who was diagnosed with FM more than seven years ago knows that having a history of more than three months of pain in all four quadrants of the body plus tenderness in 11 of 18 specific points were the previous, very specific criteria for diagnosis. That began to change soon after publication of the first edition of Tender Points. What is now recognized by the medical community and what many sufferers always knew is that sometimes very common additional symptoms can be even more debilitating than the always present pain and fatigue. Now that the ACR has expanded the basis for diagnosis, many more people will be correctly diagnosed and understood and will be given the help they need to deal with this often life-altering illness.

When the first edition of this book was written, FM had just been redefined as a neurologic rather than a rheumatologic illness. Since then it's been commonly referred to as a central nervous system disorder or "central sensitization". However, because the pain is mainly felt in the muscles and joints, rheumatologists continue to treat it.

Most recently, researchers are questioning whether FM could be an immune disorder. Although many questions remain unanswered, many advances have been made. For one thing, FM is now recognized as a separate entity as opposed to its previous designation as a syndrome (a collection of unrelated symptoms).

As explained in the first edition of this book, I am not a healthcare professional. However, more than half a century of symptoms and extensive research have given me "experiential expertise" that constitute the basis for writing this book. My purpose is not to give medical advice. For that, I have included the names of books written by experts in the field of FM that I have found most informative and easy to understand. (See Appendix A.)

My suggestion is that anyone who is newly diagnosed should read at least one of the books in the "About Fibromyalgia" section of the Appendix (or another book written by a medical professional who specializes in fibromyalgia) to learn the basics of the illness.

My purpose is to be your mentor, to prevent you from making some of the same mistakes I've made. Please use the information contained herein as one tool in deciding for yourself what your best course of action may be.

As described by a reviewer of the first edition of Tender Points: A Fibromyalgia Memoir, this book is "a how-to guide written by someone who has already lived the how-not-to version". If there is a central theme to the experiences I describe, it is that the outcome obtained from any new therapy you try may be woefully different from what you were expecting. Reading this book may save you time, money and effort and inspire you to explore new treatments you hadn't yet considered.

Although each case of FM is unique, I'm certain you'll see yourself on many of the following pages. Whether you're newly diagnosed or painfully familiar with FM, we share many symptoms as well as a common goal. Namely, we all would like to feel better and lead more normal lives.

Great strides are being made toward that goal every day. Many sufferers have found alternative therapies that are effective for them. With time and patience, you may find one or several that are effective for you.

New drugs are being approved at an unprecedented rate. Stem cell therapy is making great progress. A cure is becoming more likely every day. However, until one is found, please consider me a member of your personal support group, and use this book as a guide to living a more productive, less painful life.

To FM Support Group Leaders:

My hope is that this book (with its discussion questions at the end of each chapter) can simplify the job of the FM support group leader. Having been one of you myself, I'm aware that programming is an always present challenge. Without a specific topic for each meeting, too often the tone of a meeting becomes very negative. Attendees can leave feeling discouraged or frustrated rather than supported by the other members. Please consider using my chapters as a starting point for discussions, and make use of the questions provided at the end of each chapter to prompt participation.

Chapter 1

You've Got What?

Many people have never heard of fibromyalgia (FM), even though the National Fibromyalgia & Chronic Pain Association (FMCPA) estimates that 10 million Americans (four times more women than men) are affected. Even with the proliferation of television advertisements for Lyrica, Cymbalta, and Savella (the first 3 drugs approved by the FDA specifically for the treatment of fibromyalgia) some people are still unfamiliar with the illness.

Fibromyalgia is a chronic disease; that is, it's a condition that develops and perhaps worsens or improves over an extended period of time. It is not an acute condition and does not come on suddenly such as a broken bone or a heart attack. However, acute conditions, if left untreated, may develop into chronic conditions such as FM.

The most common symptoms of FM are widespread pain, extreme fatigue, sleep disorders and cognitive difficulties. In addition, many sufferers also have:

- IBS - Irritable Bowel Syndrome, aka spastic colon, characterized by severe abdominal pain, bloating, diarrhea and/or constipation or both.

- TMJ - Temporomandibular Joint Disorder - an aching pain in the jaw joint often accompanied by a crunching sound when chewing.
- Urinary frequency, aka irritable bladder.
- Numbness and tingling of the hands and feet.
- Headaches - often migraines.
- Intolerance to cold and/or heat.
- Anxiety and/or depression.
- MCS - Multiple Chemical Sensitivity - including intolerance to medications, cleaning products, perfumes, atmospheric pollution, foods, food additives, etc.
- Tendonitis.
- Trigger points that cause muscle spasms of the back and extremities.
- GERD - Gastro-Esophageal Reflux Disease
- Myofascial Pain Syndrome
- Restless Leg Syndrome.

FM may strike more than one family member. However, no hereditary link has been established. People at greatest risk are those with other rheumatic diseases. Twenty to thirty percent of those with rheumatoid arthritis also develop FM, and overweight or inactive women are more prone to developing it. The reason remains unclear.

For many years FM was thought to be an inflammatory disease. This accounts for its former name of fibrositis ("fibros", meaning connective tissue, "itis" meaning inflammation). The name changed to fibromyalgia in 1990 when diagnostic criteria for the syndrome were first established. Until ten years ago I could have said with certainty that FM was a central nervous system disorder characterized by increased sensitivity to almost everything, especially to pain.

However, immunologists (among them Torrance, Ca.'s Dr. John Chia) have proposed a totally new theory. In an article published in the 2007 Journal of Clinical Pathology, Dr. Chia suggested the possibility that FM is an immune disorder caused by an enterovirus. Clinical studies are under way using gamma globulin as treatment. It seems that the more we learn about this illness the more questions are raised.

Whatever the cause, the symptoms of FM remain the same now as they've always been. The most prominent one is total body pain of at least three month's duration (with or without 11 of the 18 tender points once considered the seminal diagnosis but which are currently controversial).

During a flare (the name given to a temporary worsening of any or all of these symptoms), I have experienced most of these ailments simultaneously. On good days, I have just 4 or 5.

The causes of flares are as many and as varied as the symptoms and equally as elusive. It could be stress, over-activity, a virus or a yeast. It could also be an accident, a psychological trauma, a change in temperature or humidity, or environmental conditions. Because there is no cure, controlling this illness is dependent upon learning what things aggravate your symptoms for you and devising ways to avoid them.

There are often warning signs that a flare is imminent. Sometimes you drop things. Your hands and feet may feel colder than usual. Your muscles may twitch. You might notice an increase in fibrofog (the name given to the cloudy thinking that comes and goes with this illness), dizziness or depression. Personally, I tend to do really dumb things - like pouring boiling water into the sugar bowl instead of the teacup or discarding the portion of the bill I was supposed to pay and keeping the advertising that came in the same envelope.

Preventing flares requires being very familiar with your own body, not allowing yourself to get too tired or too cold, doing everything in moderation and pacing. If flares are occurring regularly, it could be a sign that you need to simplify your life in some way. Perhaps you need to delegate, to finally call on those people who have offered to help you in the past, or to resolve a psychological issue that is causing you unusual stress. Or it may be time for a visit to your physician to see if a change in medication might be in order.

Many more women than men have been diagnosed with FM. The prevalence of women patients has been estimated by the NFMCPA at between 75 and 90 percent of the total. As early as 2001 Dr. Mohammad B. Yunus, a recognized expert in the field of fibromyalgia and a professor of medicine at the University of Illinois College of Medicine, postulated the reason for the discrepancy. He described an imbalance of chemicals in the brains of FM patients that play an important role in this disorder. In a paper published in '01 in Current Rheumatology Reports, Yunus called FM a neurochemical disease. He stated that people with FM have more than the normal amount of substance P, a pain-signaling neurotransmitter and less than the normal amount of serotonin, a pain-inhibiting neurotransmitter. He went on to say that some genes make people more susceptible to pain. Hormones, especially estrogen, lessen the pain threshold.

In 2002, a study done by Dr. Robert Bennett and published in Arthritis & Rheumatism (Vol. 46) reported that 20 women with FM showed they had a defect in growth hormone secretion. After being given a drug to reverse this condition, their symptoms improved. Further research is needed to verify whether the lack of growth hormone contributes to the development of FM.

As for the men, our culture teaches them to be tough, to just "suck it up". Many resist seeing healthcare professionals who could diagnose them and help treat their symptoms. This lack of reporting also contributes to the discrepancy in gender diagnosis.

Although there is no cure for fibromyalgia, there are many therapies that do bring relief. The best news about FM is that it is not a degenerative disease. It will not get progressively worse to the point where it will kill you. However, I must confess that the older I get the more difficult it has become to tolerate the symptoms. In general, flares tend to erupt more easily and last longer. As a result, daily preventive measures have become absolutely essential to maintaining my quality of life. These measures include regular exercise (both mental and physical), a healthy diet, pacing, and resting even before feeling tired. For me, a born multi-tasker, this last is by far the most difficult. I've also learned to be more aware of my body in an effort to thwart off symptoms before they develop. I find that prevention is far easier than recuperation.

Discussion Questions:

> *What are your most troubling symptoms?*
> *How do you recognize that a flare is about to occur?*
> *How do you describe your illness to people who haven't heard of it?*

Chapter 2

Doctor, Doctor

C hances are that a rheumatologist made or confirmed your diagnosis of fibromyalgia. General Practitioners (GP's) have historically been reluctant to make the diagnosis because of the very specific location of tender points - the criteria that had initially been essential for diagnosis. Rheumatologists receive special training in locating these points that GP's do not.

Now that the diagnostic criteria has been expanded, there may be fewer referrals to rheumatologists for verification, and more people with fibromyalgia may be diagnosed correctly. Several alternatives for diagnosis have been proposed, mostly based on a past history of additional common symptoms such as IBS (irritable bowel syndrome), cognitive difficulties, fatigue, etc in addition to pain in all four quadrants for at least six months.

One proposal under consideration is that a diagnosis could be made as simply as by having a patient complete two forms, either in or out of a doctor's office, no examination required at all. A diagnosis reached in this manner would not be valid for clinical purposes but could be used for research. That's the "not so good" news. The better news is that additional symptoms such a cognitive difficulties, unrefreshed sleep, and fatigue are also considered significant findings for fibromyalgia today. In the event that a patient has less than the previously required 11 of 18 tender points, a diagnosis of fibromyalgia could still be made. A great deal of controversy reigns over this topic. As of this writing any official amendment to the American College of Rheumatology's 1990 diagnostic criteria remains provisional.

One bit of good news is that research on FM has greatly expanded in recent years. A study done at the Albany Medical Center in Albany, New York showed that small skin biopsies revealed excessive sensory nerve fibers in the hands of fibromyalgia patients. This finding could be used as a future basis of diagnosing the disease or for developing new drugs to treat it in the future.

A diagnostic test for FM has been developed Dr. Bruce Gillis of Epicgenetics in conjunction with the University of Illinois. Dr. Gillis is another proponent of the theory of FM as an immune disorder. His multi-year study of 200 FM patients indicated abnormal white blood cells that affect protein molecules called chemokines and cytokines in FM patients. Although the test has been shown to be 95% effective, its price tag of $700 may prevent it from being embraced by the medical community any time soon. Without an effective treatment available, there is little incentive for insurance companies or individuals to spend this sum of money to confirm a diagnosis.

A small but exciting study done at Ohio State University is scheduled to be published in a monthly journal called Analyst. Dr. Tony Buffington, a veterinarian, was using an infrared microscope to study interstitial cystitis (IC), a condition common to cats as well as to humans. He recognized that IC patients often suffered from FM as well and later discovered a combination of amino acids that are specific to FM. This could lead to an inexpensive blood test for diagnosing FM in the future.

With the influx of funding and interest in the disease, it appears there will be a definitive test for FM some time soon. The problem remains as to what to do once you've been diagnosed with a disease that has no cure. Is there a reason to continue seeing a specialist? The answer to that question is not the same for everyone. In some cases, you absolutely MUST. In others cases, a GP can be just as helpful.

Typically, you need medical care for FM if and when your symptoms worsen or when a new symptom appears. If your medications have become ineffective you may wish to try something new or different. My experience has been that rheumatologists (and physical medicine doctors known as physiatrists) are more familiar with the performance of drugs that treat FM symptoms simply because they have more patients who use them. However, if your GP, internist or neurologist happens to have a considerable number of patients with FM, he/she may be equally or more qualified.

Thus far, only three prescription drugs have been approved by the FDA for use in fibromyalgia. They are Lyrica, Cymbalta and Savella. Three more are in the pipeline that are currently used to treat other illnesses but are being tested for effectiveness in FM as well. They are Nothera, Seroquel and Edronax. If you haven't already tried them, perhaps one of these may be helpful for you now or at some time in the future. I know several people who claim to be greatly improved with the use of Lyrica and/or Cymbalta. Unfortunately, none of the three worked for me.

Here's an interesting fact you won't find in any medical book. Even though FM patients comprise as much as half of many rheumatology practices, they are the poor stepchildren of the specialty. The reason is that our aging population has resulted in more arthritis sufferers than ever before, creating a severe shortage of rheumatologists. As a result, many practices are routinely overbooked. Their focus, necessarily, is on the patient in acute pain, like many rheumatoid arthritis (RA) patients. When you've been one of them as I have (I happen to have RA in addition to fibromyalgia), you can appreciate this bitter fact. Chronic pain sufferers, such as FM patients, often take a back seat when appointments are scheduled. It is also possible that because FM has been labeled a neurological disorder for the past several years rheumatologists may be reluctant to include new FM patients in their practice.

Is this unfair? You bet it is! After years of suffering and having no diagnosis at all, you've finally arrived at a specialist who understands your illness and recognizes the fact that you are truly ill. But now you're being treated like a second-class citizen. Is it the doctor's fault? Not at all. There are only so many patients that can be seen in a day. The sickest must come first. I didn't understand this situation early in my illness. As a result, I labeled several excellent doctors as "uncaring" or even "incompetent." In actuality, they were merely overworked.

While we're on the topic of specialists: Many insurance plans require a referral from your Primary Care Provider (PCP) before you can visit a specialist (i.e., a rheumatologist or neurologist). His staff may even schedule the appointment for you. Please don't be misled into thinking that the day and time of that appointment is written in stone. If it's inconvenient for you, just call the specialist's office when you get home and ask to reschedule. The important part is the referral; the day and time of the appointment are secondary.

If you are told to wait for a call from a specialist's office to schedule an appointment, don't do it. That's right. Don't wait. Have that number in hand before you leave your primary care doctor's office, and make that call right away. The wait for an appointment can be several weeks long, and those several weeks don't begin until you speak to someone on the phone. If you're told by the specialist's office that they have no referral for you, don't hesitate to call back to your primary care doctor's office to give them a little nudge to get it done.

Depending on the type of insurance you have, a pre-authorization request may also be required before you can see a specialist. This may be a bit more complicated because it requires your doctor's office to interact with your insurance company.

The first step is that your doctor's office contacts your insurance company. Next, the insurance company considers the request and transmits its answer back to your doctor's office. Then your doctor's office notifies you - either by phone, mail or email. Only after you have this authorization can make your own appointment with the specialist. If everyone is doing his job, the process can take as little as 24 hours. More commonly, it drags on for weeks.

Again, don't let that happen. Be proactive. Here's how you can speed up the process:

- Call your doctor's office 24 hours after your appointment to ask about the status of your authorization request. If they haven't contacted your insurance company yet, this will be a gentle reminder for them to do so.
- Call your doctor's office 2 days later to see if they've received the authorization back from the insurance company. They will tell you they have not, (even though they probably have) but it will urge them to sort through their incoming emails or faxes to see if it's there.

- Call back the next day and ask the same question.
- If the answer is still "no", call the insurance company and ask to speak to the person in charge of specialist authorizations.
- If the answer is "yes", ask your doctor's office staff not to mail the authorization to you but to fax or email it to the specialist's office you wish to see.
- Call the specialist for an appointment. Mention that your doctor's office has sent them the authorization from your insurance company. If they haven't received it, they will know who to call.
- If the referral you receive is with a physician you don't wish to see, call the insurance company. They really don't care who you see, they only care whether the paper work is in order. In many instances, they will be happy to refer you to any physician in that field who is in their network.

The lesson to be learned here is to be persistent. The painful truth is that no one cares about your medical problems except you. You must learn to be your own advocate.

Another thing to keep in mind insurance-wise is that an HMO does not require you to jump through hoops to get from a primary care doctor to a specialist. Sadly, people with fibromyalgia are known to have such varied symptoms that specialist visits are almost inevitable. In addition, there is no annoying paper work. Yes, you are limited to doctors in their network, so be sure to choose wisely if you're considering an HMO. But also consider that openings for physicians at HMO's are very sought after these days which means that you're quite likely to receive excellent care. Many of the brightest, most qualified young physicians are vying for these jobs because of the lifestyle it affords them. For a young doctor with a young family, the hours and on-call requirements of an HMO are more conducive to a normal home life than being affiliated with a private practice that requires frequent on-call hours. HMO's also offer the advantage of having all their doctors electronically connected. This can be especially helpful when a patient has a complicated history as many FM patients do. Additionally, in my own personal experience, their referrals are accomplished much more smoothly than with a non-HMO insurance plan.

Even though a diagnosis doesn't get you cured, it is a starting point for treating the symptoms. Because every case is very different there are no standard treatments. Finding what works for you can be as challenging as arriving at a correct diagnosis. Yes, you should work with your doctor for the best results. However, it is a great advantage if you keep yourself as well informed as possible. Helping yourself feel better is largely a process of trial and error, requiring a great deal of time and patience.

We all have a tendency to want to unload all our symptoms all at once to any new physician we happen to see. If it's one who is particularly knowledgeable about the illness that ails us, the temptation is even greater. My advice is to limit your complaints to only 3 per visit. This way you won't overwhelm your provider and are more likely to receive more knowledgeable, more effective treatment. Here are some guidelines you might want to consider for your next physician's visit.

DO

Provide accurate information – only facts, not feelings
Write down your questions before you go
Bring someone with you (another set of ears)
Be diplomatic, yet assertive
Do your research before you go
Ask questions about the treatment prescribed

DON'T

Arrive ready for battle
Be long winded about your suffering
Expect your doctor to be a therapist

As to the question of whether or not you need to continue to see a specialist after you've been diagnosed: Once your symptoms have been stabilized, your primary care doctor can usually follow you along for routine care as well as a rheumatologist can - with just a few exceptions.

One exception might be a need for physical therapy (PT). Depending upon your insurance coverage, a PT referral must come from a specialist. I, for one, have found PT to be the very best treatment for several of my ailments including Myofascial Pain Syndrome. Because I'm unable to tolerate any of the medications available to treat this painful symptom, I've had to turn to alternative therapies. Unfortunately, acupuncture, acupressure, reflexology and aromatherapy were all ineffective. The only relief I've found is with the exercises prescribed by my physical therapist. I've also been referred to PT at various times for leg and knee strengthening. My legs sometimes buckle and I've fallen down stairs more than once. PT exercises, if used on a continuous basis can be an enormous help with these and additional muscle issues that commonly plague FM sufferers.

Another exception is for treatment of acute pain, although with our nation's current opioid crisis this has become a sticky issue. A rheumatologist may be more willing to prescribe an opiate if you need it - for severe flares or for episodes of breakthrough pain. In many states, narcotic prescriptions written by GP's and family practice physicians are so over-regulated that the doctors have been bullied into under-prescribing opiates - even for their patients in acute pain. They may refer you to a pain specialist instead. Some states have recently established guidelines for physicians for prescribing opiates. Unfortunately, chronic pain patients have not been properly considered in these diagnoses. There is a great need for effective pain relief in a form that doesn't include addictive medications that can destroy a patient's organs. Cannabis holds great promise for the future. To date, so little research has been done that it's still considered dangerous and experimental.

The third situation for which you definitely need to have a rheumatologist is if you have filed or are considering filing for disability in the future. During this nasty process all your doctors will be required to complete reports describing your illness and how it affects your ability to work. Insurance companies (and the Social Security Administration in particular) seem to value the opinion of a rheumatologist over that of a general practitioner - even one who has known you your entire life.

Let me assure you that your rheumatologist will not enjoy doing the paperwork involved in a disability case, so try to be as helpful as you can be. The form located in Appendix C is a good place to begin. The form may also be found on my website at www.fmspubs.com. My suggestion is to complete the form the best you can before any appointment, bring two copies with you, and then discuss what you've written with your doctor. He will appreciate your effort and will use the information on the form as a basis for his report.

Regardless of his/her specialty, a doctor who is reasonably available, well informed, and open-minded is your best option. My definition of "reasonably available" is a same-day appointment for an acute ailment, 3-5 days for a routine matter. I define well informed as a doctor who knows more about my illness than I do. I define open-minded as being willing to listen to and to discuss new information I've found without dismissing it as being irrelevant because I found it on the internet. Open-minded is also giving the patient credit for knowing his own body as well as (if not better than) the doctor does.

Good doctors are out there, and they are worth the effort it takes to find them. Ask friends and relatives, acquaintances who work in the medical field, people who also have chronic illnesses. Most people are happy to honestly tell you how they feel about their doctors.

The truth is that when it comes to fibromyalgia, even the best doctors only know the facts. They don't know the nitty gritty; how it changes your life, alters your goals, destroys your dreams. They haven't had to adapt their lives to the challenges we face each day, so they have no advice to give on that topic. Medical schools don't teach them this. For this kind of information, you need advice from someone who's been there and can understand, someone like me, or another fellow sufferer.

Two notable exceptions to this rule that I'm familiar with are Dr. Paul St. Amand, and Dr. Jacob Teitelbaum. Dr. St. Amand (an endocrinologist) routinely treats FM patients with guafenesin, the active ingredient in Robitussin. He claims that it is responsible for having cured his own FM. It is an option worth considering. It has worked for many people (including two that I know personally), although it didn't happen to work for me.

After having lost a year of medical school because of Chronic Fatigue Syndrome (a close relative of FM), Dr. Jacob Teitelbaum has gone on to become a leading CFIDS (chronic fatigue and immune dysfunction) clinician and researcher. His excellent book, From Fatigued to Fantastic, emphasizes the importance of analyzing and treating nutritional deficiencies.

Regardless of your doctor's specialty, recognize that he/she is only one member of your healthcare team. Hopefully, there will be others on your team as well. There may be a physical therapist, a nutritionist, a massage therapist, a yoga instructor, a psychiatrist, a psychologist or social worker, a meditation coach, an acupuncturist, a chiropractor, etc.

Remember that the most important member of your healthcare team is you. Learn all you can. Try new things. Talk to people. With time and patience you will find what works for you. You can lead the life you were meant to live. You just need to learn how to do it on your own terms, in your own way, and be comfortable with it.

Believe anything is possible and it is!

Discussion Questions:

> *How long did it take for you to be diagnosed?*
> *What qualities do you appreciate most in your doctor(s)?*
> *Do you routinely see a primary care doc for your FM or do you see a rheumatologist – and why?*

Chapter 3

Do Your Homework

You can help your doctors to help you by keeping yourself informed. With the avalanche of information available on the internet today, it can be overwhelming to keep up with the latest developments as well as with the most informative websites to visit. The challenge is to sort through it all and to know what is accurate and up-to-date.

The natural temptation is to believe everything you read on the internet, but here are a few words of caution. Be wary of information found at web addresses ending in ".com." Even though they may contain some good information, their primary purpose is "com"merce. In other words, they want to sell you something. Websites ending with ".org", ".edu", or ".gov" denote an affiliation with an unbiased institution such as a non-profit group, a university or a government agency. You are more likely to get accurate information from sites like these.

Many of the publications and websites I once relied upon for legitimate information have been discontinued as the symptoms of the administrators (many of whom were patients themselves) became too severe for them to continue their efforts. One such recent loss was the Fibromyalgia Network and its wonderful newsletter.

This quarterly publication described the newest research being conducted on fibromyalgia in laymans' terms and accurately reported the results. Unfortunately, its editor, Kristin Thorsen, became too ill to continue.

Even the National Fibromyalgia Association (the NFA) had to completely reorganize after its director, Lynn Matallana, was involved in a serious accident that required major surgery. The loss of the NFA was a tremendous blow to the FM community, given the wonderful work that organization has done on behalf of FM patients worldwide. Portions of the work previously done by the NFA have been absorbed by the National Fibromyalgia and Chronic Pain Association (NFmCPA). Their current website is fmcpaware.org, although a name change for the site appears to be forthcoming.

The most current, accurate and up-to-date website I know is Fibromyalgia News Today (for which I currently write a weekly column entitled "Tender Points".) Dedicated patient authors keep themselves informed about new developments in the field and share their information and their experiences with their readers. Each article has a comments column where people share their thoughts about the content. I have found writing this column to be hugely rewarding as I receive feedback from people all over the world who have opinions to add or additional topics to discuss.

PatientsLikeMe.com is another site that has existed for several years and addresses many diseases in addition to FM. It contains valuable tools to help patients track the progress of their own illness. Despite the fact that the site is sponsored by a major pharmaceutical company, I do recommend this one. Being the cynic I am, I'm suspicious that the site's ultimate goal is to convince me that I need a drug that I don't. However, this hasn't happened yet. So I still check in with their chat room from time to time to see if any topics of interest to me are being discussed. Much like a support group, the conversations there have led me to explore new treatment options that have proven helpful and that I have shared with others.

If an advertisement for a treatment or a product says it's been scientifically studied, there are sources where you can verify that fact. One of them is www.PubMed.com. Here you can search a database maintained by the National Library of Medicine. It contains information on double-blind studies that have been peer-reviewed and publicized in journals such as Rheumatology, The New England Journal of Medicine, and the Journal of the American Medical Association. Unlike other articles found on the internet, results of studies found here are almost certain to impress your physician.

Even if a study appears to be legitimate, it's never a good idea to rely on the results of a single study. Rather, read all you can wherever you can. A good place to start is with one of the books listed in Appendix A.

A word of caution: Discuss your findings with your doctor before you invest any money in a so-called "cure." If it sounds too good to be true, chances are that it is. However, having taken the appropriate steps to verify the information, I say, "If it won't hurt you or hurt your budget, try it." People have been helped by some of the strangest things!

One thing to keep in mind is that everyone's body is different. Something that helps one person won't necessarily help you and vice versa. I knew a woman who swore that a magnetic mattress pad completely cured her pain. I tried one with a money-back guarantee and awoke with severe pain all over my body after the first night. The second night was no better. I promptly received a refund. Other people I know swear by the Cuddledown feather bed. All it did for me was to make me sneeze. Again, the full price of the product (approx. $500) was refunded - no questions asked. Because there was no risk to my wallet or my body, I felt both items were worth a try. My search continues.

Another good source of information is a support group. (More on that topic in another chapter) Not only can you learn a great deal from the other members, but most groups routinely invite knowledgeable speakers. Even if you don't learn anything that's useful to you, you'll have a chance to vent your frustrations in a setting where everyone understands them. And you'll feel better about yourself for having taken an active role in assisting in your own well-being.

Discussion Questions:

> *What is your primary source of information about FM?*
> *How receptive is your doctor to the information you bring to him about FM?*
> *Have you learned anything recently that you found useful in reducing your symptoms?*

Chapter 4

Growing Up with Fibro

L ooking back, it's clear to me that I've had fibromyalgia all my life. Everyone raved at what a good baby I was. I think I was just too exhausted to make a fuss, even then!

As a small child I regularly had trouble sleeping. My mother's advice to "Just go back to bed and lay there with your eyes closed" didn't help one bit. Instead, as the hours passed, my body would grow stiff and achy. Eventually, I learned to focus on the pain (my earliest experience with meditation), and would drift off to sleep that way. Later, I read by flashlight under the covers. I was often awake after midnight, leaving me tired and sleepy all the next day. Although I did well in school, I was always exhausted when I got home.

I never had as much energy as the other kids, preferring board games and paper dolls to active games like tag or softball. I was one of the original couch potatoes - except in the summer - which I spent at the city pool. This was the only relief I had from the heat in the days before air conditioning. In addition, the buoyancy of my body in the water made it the one place I could keep up with the other kids.

Outside of the swimming pool, summers were pretty miserable for me. My mother always insisted I "eat something" even if it was over 90 degrees in the house. With my intolerance to heat, vomiting after dinner was not an unusual occurrence. I fainted and fell off the risers during my 8th grade graduation ceremony held outdoors on a balmy 85-degree day.

If I complained about the total body pain I was experiencing, our family doctor attributed it to "growing pains." Aspirin was prescribed which caused additional pain in my very sensitive stomach. At the age of 10, what I referred to as my "Midol Misery" began. Every month, several hours before my menstrual period started, I became one big mass of muscle tension. I felt slightly manic, like I wanted to scream for no reason at all. Physically, it felt like I had two internal rubber bands, one connected from my abdomen to my toes, the other from my abdomen to my fingers. Each one was being pulled tighter and tighter. My toes curled, my fists clenched, I would sweat profusely and moan involuntarily. No amount of Midol or anything else relieved this agony. Only sleep (even if only for a few minutes) would relax the tension and the telltale sign would appear in my underwear upon awakening.

Every month I went through the same thing. Suffering too badly to be embarrassed, I would get excused from class to go see the nurse. I would tell her I had "cramps" rather than try to explain my actual symptoms, get excused from school, and drag myself home in tears. After a short nap, the flow would begin and I'd be fine until the next cycle, anywhere from 18 to 45 days from the start of the previous episode. During that entire time I fervently prayed that the next episode would occur at night or on a weekend. Then I'd be closer to my bed.

For a long time I thought all young girls felt the way I did. When I finally realized how different my monthly experience was, I reluctantly allowed my mother to take me to a doctor, even though I was terrified he might perform the dreaded "internal exam". But I was desperate. I would have done absolutely anything not to have to suffer that way again.

This was my first experience with trying to describe what was wrong with me to a member of the medical community. It was actually good practice for when the next bizarre fibromyalgia symptoms appeared. Unfortunately, no amount of explaining could make the kindly old doc understand my problem. I'm not sure there was anything he could have done for me even if he did. Disappointing as that was, I was more relieved that no "internal exam" had been performed.

What the doctor told my mother (as if I wasn't even in the room) was that in time I'd learn to live with "having cramps" and being a woman. He was wrong. What I had was never "cramps," and I never did learn to live with whatever it was that I had. I experienced this "Midol Misery" every single month until I began taking birth control pills shortly before marriage at the age of 20. Had they been available in 1957, birth control pills begun at age 10 might have saved me a world of hurt.

It wasn't until I attended a fibromyalgia seminar when I was 47 years old that I learned my premenstrual symptoms had not been unique. Muscle tension of this sort is actually quite common for fibromites. Several women present at that meeting described the exact same manic, sweaty feeling, accompanied by clenching of their hands and feet. In menstruation, as in so many other things, FM bodies respond differently than most other bodies do.

At pajama parties, I was the one who always fell asleep while the others were eating midnight pizza. Fortunately, these events were usually held on Fridays, as I would be a total zombie for the next two days. Then, because of the lack of sleep, a sore throat would develop, followed by a stuffy head and usually a cold sore or two. These symptoms often progressed to bronchitis with a high fever, requiring a trip to the doctor and a penicillin shot. Because the resulting illnesses so often led to my missing days from school, my mother eventually forbade me to attend sleepovers. I was devastated. It was a fate worse than death to a teen-aged girl!

In college, I was the only one in my social circle who couldn't abide going to bars or fraternity parties. The loud music would actually cause my ears to ring and my head to ache. And even though I was an occasional smoker myself at the time, being in a densely smoke-filled environment where you could barely see across the room, would cause my chest to hurt and make me cough for the next several days. I was fortunate to usually have a boyfriend who sympathized with my plight, so the two of us would go to a local burger joint or the library instead.

Not all young adults with FM are as fortunate as I was. Many are labeled unsociable because of their inability to tolerate the conditions of smoky parties and loud bands. They lead isolated lives in their dormitories or at home. The bright side is that they are likely to earn excellent grades because they have little else to do but study. As a result, many become successful in their endeavors. This might sound like an advantage to an adult, but it's a very lonely life for a 19-yr-old student.

Fortunately this situation is changing. Juvenile fibromyalgia is now a recognized disorder. Similar to adult fibromyalgia, it is characterized by total body muscular pain, with fatigue, sleep and mood issues as well. Estimates by the Mayo Clinic are that juvenile onset F affects between two and six percent of school children, most commonly girls between the ages of 3 and 15.

Discussion Questions:

> *At what age did you develop the symptoms of FM?*
> *How soon did you receive a diagnosis?*
> *Were there any precipitating factor(s) like a virus or an accident?*

Chapter 5

Fibromyalgia Dating

We would all like to have a healthy partner to help us through the bad times. However, given the choice of living with someone who has as many symptoms as I have or living alone, I'd prefer to live alone. That being said, there is also such a thing as a partner who is too healthy. Many people who've never had medical issues have a hard time relating to us. They would like us to "Just Say Yes" and don't understand why we "Just Say No."

Dating is a challenge under any circumstances, but especially so when you have fibromyalgia - even on the good days. You're constantly choosing between revealing how you really feel or how you wish you felt. You want to be honest without coming across as sickly. In many ways, you're not. You're perfectly capable of doing lots of the things that most other people do – although you may need to do less or do it with modifications. With any luck you'll get past the first few encounters with a new acquaintance without having to unveil your limitations.

We are fortunate to now have the Internet as a tool in our search for a mate. It's no longer necessary to spend evenings at a singles bar trying to look available. Legitimate services like Match.com, E-Harmony and many others bring together many lucky couples. I became a widow a year before Match entered the scene, and I was one of the pioneers in using its services when it debuted. To say it was frightening at first is an understatement. However, after a few successful encounters, I considered it a great adventure. I met many interesting men as well as some of their friends. I got to participate in activities I may never have done. All in all, it was a positive experience for me.

My one suggestion before going the internet route is to open a new email account to use exclusively for purposes of internet dating. Be sure this account doesn't have any portion of your last name or phone number in it. Communicating by email is a must before meeting anyone in person. The last thing you want is to give the account name you regularly use to a stranger who might turn into a pain in the computer – or to a faker or a hacker who could track you down from information in your email address.

The nearly limitless supply of people available (remember the Internet is international) forces you to assess what things are really important to you in a relationship. After a few disastrous meetings, you learn to ask very specific questions ahead of time, quickly ruling out those you have absolutely no interest in getting to know. Once you've exchanged a few e-mails, I suggest a phone call or two. But, you call him, not the other way around. Never divulge your phone number or your last name to anyone before you've had a face-to-face opportunity to make an assessment.

Keeping in mind that the person you are hoping to meet is very different from the person I was seeking, here are a few of the questions I found useful when I played the internet dating game. Keep in mind that you don't want to ask questions with "yes " or "no" answers. Give your new acquaintance an opportunity to tell you about him/herself.

- What's your favorite way to spend a rainy day?
- Tell me about the best vacation you ever had.
- How much reading do you do? Who's your favorite author?
- What's your favorite restaurant? Your favorite meal there?
- What are you favorite foods? Which ones do you prepare for yourself?
- What type of music do you enjoy?
- How do you feel about ballroom dancing? Ever take lessons? Would you be willing to?
- Describe a typical day with your children/grandchildren (depending on age).

The last thing you want to discuss is your illness. Although it's far easier to explain your limitations in advance than it is to think of an excuse on the spot, it's not something you want to do before the third date. It's better to keep the conversation light and generic. Be sure to discuss topics you know a lot about and enjoy. With any luck, you'll discover that the other person also knows about and enjoys discussing it. Now you have a basis for your relationship! Take every opportunity to show who you really are - anything other than the aching, exhausted bag of bones you often feel like.

The purpose of the answers to the questions you ask, of course, is to rule out the people who aren't interested in the things that interest you. My list evolved over time, and yours will, too. The answers to your questions will be a good indication of your compatibility, but the absolute best test is seeing where and how that person lives – which won't happen until you've spent some time together. The reason this is so important is that PEOPLE DON'T CHANGE.

If a person tosses his clothes on the floor and leaves dirty dishes on the coffee table now, don't think that this behavior will change in the future. If the screen door is hanging off its hinges and the paint is peeling off his house, that's an excellent indication of what your future home together might look like. If you're not happy living that way, your relationship is doomed.

One technique to get to see how the other person lives is to offer to pick him up for a second or third daytime date. You won't need to go any further than the front doorway to get the idea. You'll know in an instant whether or not to go any further. Remember everyone has different standards.

Never give out your phone number until you've met this stranger and are certain you would like to see him/her again. Rather, ask for his phone number by e-mail, and you call him from someplace other than your home phone. If you wish to meet him after you've had a phone conversation or two, arrange to do so in a safe and public place. A coffee shop is a good choice.

So, you've met several times casually, you liked each other's company, and now he's coming to pick you up for a real date. So far, so good. You open the door and your eyes begin to water. Achoo! He wasn't wearing this cloud of cologne when you met before. Why is he wearing it now? How do you tell this man to go home and wash his face? You don't. This is the point you begin to get real, but gently. You tell him you're so very sorry, but that you have many "allergies" and that his cologne must contain one of them. This is not yet time for a tutorial about Multiple Chemical Sensitivity. His reaction will be an opportunity for you to see how he reacts to what would be a common occurrence were you to have a relationship.

A week later you meet at a restaurant for lunch on a rainy day. Already seated, you see him arrive with a pretty bouquet of roses and eucalyptus. The warning light goes off in your brain. As he approaches, the countdown begins. 10, 9, 8... At about 7 your eyes are squinting. ...6, 5. At 4 the first tears begin dripping down your face. 3,2,1 "Achoo!!" Flowers now in hand, you're actually weeping and becoming nauseous from the scent. Tears are dripping steadily, staining your new silk blouse.

Could you feign a swoon? Why are you doing this to yourself? You could be curled up on your couch with a good book and a glass of wine or a cup of herbal tea! The reason is because you don't want to be alone on your couch with your book and your wine or your tea for the rest of your life!

So you say, "Remember those allergies I told you about last week? I'm afraid I'm allergic to many flowers as well, actually anything with a scent. I'm so sorry. They're really very beautiful". "No, I'm sorry," he says, as he slinks away and presents the bouquet to a pair of grateful elderly ladies lunching across the room. (One point for him!)

Regardless of how well he handled it, this is not an ego builder, and it requires some first-aid (assuming he returns to the table). My advice? Keep it light. Laugh at your foibles. Tell him about a similar experience and exaggerate the hell out of it. Think of anything else the least bit amusing that's happened in your life as a result of having MCS. Lie if you must. Go for the laugh when nothing else works. It's not dishonest; it's just the lighter side of your life and a preview of what's to come.

If he's not disenchanted at this point, from here on, let your problems become apparent, a little at a time. Without being dramatic about it, you need to prepare him for what a relationship with you would be like. He's had some time to get to know you. He obviously enjoys your company or he wouldn't be present for the second or third time. If he's really interested, he'll probably admit to some problems of his own. If it all goes south and you never hear from him again, consider yourself blessed. You've just saved yourself a lot of time and effort you could have used to meet someone else who could become your life partner.

Attitude is everything when using internet dating. If you think of it as an adventure, as a fun excuse to get out of the house and meet a new friend, your chances of success are much greater than if you're putting your hopes and dreams into finding your mate for life. That kind of pressure can ruin any potential relationship. I can guarantee you one thing for sure. You will definitely have some unusual experiences.

For example, I once drove 50 miles to meet a man I'd chatted with online for months. Because it was winter in central New York, and because we were geographically separated by more than an hour, we'd extended our emailing while awaiting better weather. In the interim, we'd exchanged photos, family backgrounds, and life histories, finding we had much in common. I had great hope for this meeting and even for a possible relationship.

Finally, we met for brunch at a restaurant located an equal distance from each of us. All went well until he smiled broadly at me across the table and revealed a full set of gold teeth! Perhaps his mouth was a fashion statement in the Baltic country from which he came, but it was shockingly unattractive to me. That brunch may have been the longest hour I've ever spent in my life. As soon as I got home I checked the photos he'd sent. His mouth was firmly closed in every one.

If on-line dating sites aren't your thing, there are other places to meet your Prince Charming. One place I discovered quite by accident was a night school class I took in Statistics. More than half the class consisted of policemen who were doing what I was doing at that time - expanding an Associates degree into a Bachelor's degree in preparation for a promotion. There were at least a dozen young, attractive, goal-oriented men in that class, and they were nearly all single – allowing them time to attend night classes rather than reading bedtime stories and tucking in the kids. I happened to be married at the time and nearly 20 years older than most of them were! Telling my younger, single friends about my fellow classmates went a long way toward boosting admission to that college the following semester.

Courses in sports of any kind are another great place to meet men and to make friends with like-minded women. Take a class in anything you've always wanted to try. The great thing is that anyone you meet there will be a beginner just like you. Try Scottish dancing, sculpting, golf or fly-fishing. Take a chance! Remember, you only live once.

Get involved in something that interests you. It could be a church group, a volunteer group or politics. If you meet someone there, you will immediately have something in common. That's the first step toward building any relationship.

Above all, don't despair. Beginning a year after my husband died, I dated for nearly nine years before I met my second husband. Searching for a mate was an important goal in my life. I was determined to find a special someone, and I was willing to invest a great deal of time and effort into find the right man. Eventually I did.

Remember you're still you - with or without fibromyalgia. Your intellect hasn't been diminished by your illness, although your memory probably isn't what it used to be. Your personality was formed before you became ill. If anything, you're a better person now as a result. You know what things are really important in life. And you can recognize compassion when you see it.

If being with another person is important to you, go for it. But treat it as you would any other important objective. A half-hearted effort isn't likely to produce results. Search everywhere. Enlist all the help you can muster. You never know where Mr. Right will be. But you'll never find him if you're curled up on your couch with a book and a beverage.

Discussion Questions:

> *Have you had any experience with dating after you developed FM symptoms?*
> *Did you meet this person online or from a friend or mutual interest?*
> *What advice do you have for the rest of the group?*

Chapter 6

Having a Baby!

Although I hadn't yet been diagnosed with fibromyalgia, (There were no diagnostic criteria until 1990.) my pregnancy experience in 1969 was far from normal. For one thing, my morning sickness began the morning after I conceived. It lasted all that day, and continued for most of the entire time I carried my baby. Thankfully, he arrived six weeks early. In addition to the nausea, I was so exhausted the entire time that I lay on the couch and watched TV all day. Often, my only activity was cooking dinner for my husband - on the rare occasions when I could get past the odors of the food I was cooking. Our little apartment had dust bunnies the size of cats. I was the original couch potato.

Few studies have been done on the relationship between FM and pregnancy. The only one of note was done at Temple University in 2006. The results were not surprising. "Pregnant women with FM had a hard time functioning, felt more stiff and tired, and experienced pain in more body areas than women without FM." No surprise there!

The fact that many FM sufferers are counseled or choose not to take pain medication and anti-depressants during their pregnancy could account for the increase in symptoms. Alternative treatments such as massage, exercise, yoga, meditation and rest are all excellent substitutes which were never suggested to me at the time.

The childbirth classes I attended prepared me for labor pains (during which time you panted) with recovery time in between (during which time you took long breaths). Unfortunately, that wasn't my experience at all. Instead, I had one, intense, continuous pain which began before noon and ended in the delivery room 6:03 p.m. I scrunched up my face and pushed so hard to get the baby out that I ruptured every blood vessel in the whites of both my eyes. They were a lovely shade of crimson for the next several weeks, frightening everyone who came to see the new baby.

The good news was that my baby (Brian) was normal and healthy, although a bit jaundiced because of being born so early. The bad news was that I sank into a deep post-partum depression, another condition that had yet to be named. In addition, because he was a colicky baby, my lack of sleep worsened the state of my immune system such that I contracted every cold and flu that went around.

Before my pregnancy, my weight averaged 128 lbs. Morning sickness brought it down to 112 and baby weight increased it to 134. After giving birth, I was back down to 128 again and left the hospital wearing my pre-pregnancy clothes. A year after giving birth, I weighed 107. I wasn't trying to diet. I just didn't feel well (mentally or physically) and didn't care if I ate or not.

I was referred from specialist to specialist, finally arriving at a psychiatric clinic where they seemed to think my problem was sexual in nature. Only later did I discover that during this particular era, the field of psychiatry thought all emotional problems were sexual in nature. There were many other schools of thought, but I was truly uninformed on the topic. (This was long before research was possible via the internet.)

Also, at that time there was still an enormous stigma regarding psychotherapy. It was assumed by many that if you needed that kind of help it meant you were "crazy". In addition, psychological counseling was hugely expensive and not covered by many insurance plans. I was fortunately to be living in a city with a medical school. Their residents in the department of psychiatry saw patients on a siding fee scale, so it was affordable for me. Too embarrassed to tell my neighbor who was baby-sitting for me that I was seeing a psychiatrist, I claimed to have an ongoing urinary tract infection - ongoing for nearly 2 years! Keeping this secret just added to my misery and my feelings of isolation.

In retrospect, my emotional problems were likely the result of two conditions, both well recognized and commonly treatable today. The first, no doubt, was fibromyalgia. The second: a protracted case of post-partum depression.

Having fibromyalgia as an inexperienced young mother brought many challenges, but the worst was loneliness. We had moved to a new city 50 miles away from home just before I became pregnant. We had no family, no friends, and no babysitters. Yes, there were other young mothers in the neighborhood, but I believed in the old adage that "You have to be a friend in order to have a friend". And I was always too fatigued to make the effort. When asked to become part of a "You watch my child, then I'll watch yours" arrangement, I had to decline. As much as I wanted to participate, most days I had trouble enough caring for me and my own. I wasn't comfortable sharing my embarrassing illness with women I barely knew, so I maintained my distance.

I also think the strain and the exhaustion of having had a difficult pregnancy also took its toll on me. In truth, I believe it took me nearly two years to recover from my pregnancy. Although post-partum depression didn't have a name at that time, no name was needed to see the depression I felt.

I had a wonderful husband, but he traveled a lot on business, often being away 2 or 3 nights a week. After having driven hundreds of miles during the week, the last thing he wanted to do was to get in the car on weekends. He was happy staying home and playing with the baby. That gave me an opportunity to do something on my own, but I was usually too tired and preferred taking long naps instead. As a result, we had a very few social engagements and fewer friends. It was an unhealthy situation all around.

In addition, I was wracked with guilt. My pediatrician (the father of nine very healthy children that he had little hand in raising) was totally unsympathetic toward me and my colicky baby. He made no effort to reassure me that his screams were not the result of my inexperienced mothering.

In those days breast feeding had gone out of style. Obstetricians routinely injected new mothers with a medication to dry up their milk. On my doctor's advice, that's what I did. In retrospect, lack of breast milk certainly must have contributed to the digestive difficulties experienced by my premature baby.

My pediatrician's primary focus was to find the formula that would sooth my baby's intestines. We tried every formula on the market, from soy to lamb to beef, and on and on. None of them made the slightest difference. In the end, four months of growth and the complete development of his digestive system was the thing that ended the colic – by which time my digestive system had its own issues from the stress of it all.

Abdominal pain and diarrhea kept me up as many nights as my crying baby did. With a strong family history of colon cancer, I sought medical help each time these symptoms became severe. I underwent a lifetime's worth of sigmoidoscopies and barium enemas during my 20s. When the results routinely came back negative, I was referred for psychological help. I was analyzed from A to Z but my symptoms didn't improve. I was told to go home and relax. That was a joke! I was too exhausted to do anything BUT relax.

Fatigue was my biggest challenge. I slept every time the baby napped and sometimes when he was awake. He was always safe, either in a crib or a playpen, but I often cried whenever he cried because I didn't have the energy to pick him up. I suffered a terrific case of the "guilts".

The situation greatly improved when he was old enough to listen to stories and look at pictures. After that, reading on the couch cuddled together was how we spent our days. Even that used all the energy I had, but it was doable.

They say that every cloud has a silver lining. If that's true, then the silver lining in this situation was that my son developed an abiding love of books. I'm guessing he associated reading with the warmth and constancy of snuggling with his mother. Besides, the stories in the books were more exciting than his mundane reality.

Dr. Seuss' books were particular favorites. First the characters, then the rhymes became a part of our family. By the age of three, Brian could recite every book verbatim. Trips to the library were our special treats. We'd always leave with as many books as we could carry. A stop for ice cream on the way home completed the outing.

While filling out a college application during his junior year in High School, Brian was having difficulty selecting an author for an essay entitled, "The most influential writer in my life." Given the amount of reading he had done by then, it wasn't surprising. When asked for my suggestion, I said, "That's easy. It was Dr. Seuss!" He immediately agreed, wrote his essay and received early acceptance at Princeton University. That's what I call a silver lining!

Just as no two cases of fibromyalgia are alike, no two pregnancies are alike either. Plenty of women with FM have perfectly normal pregnancies and deliveries. Some of my FM support group members claim they felt better at that time of their lives than they ever felt before or since. So, don't expect to have problems just because I did.

Knowing the cause of my symptoms would have been a real comfort to me as a young mother, especially during the toddler years. Instead, I felt like I was just lazy, a terrible failure who could only watch as other mothers pushed their children in strollers, socializing and enjoying motherhood.

I beat myself up plenty during those years. Don't let this happen to you. Do whatever you can do, be sure your kids know you love them, and rest whenever you need to. Understand that fibromyalgia is a real illness, just as real as diabetes or epilepsy.

Accept any help that's offered, and don't hesitate to ask for what you need. Over time I've learned that if people understand you're struggling with health issues, they're very motivated to help you. Perhaps they were once in need themselves. Perhaps they have a family member who has issues and they don't live close enough to help them. Helping you may be just what they need to feel better about themselves. Your reality is what it is. Hiding it doesn't help anybody – especially you. It took me a long time to learn that people won't judge you for being ill – physically or psychologically. In fact, your honesty could be just the opening they'd been wanting in order to be able to share some problem with you as well.

Above all, don't feel guilty about asking for help. Your turn to repay the kindness will come. You will feel better in the future. Fibromyalgia has its ups and downs. You won't feel awful forever, and you won't have a baby to care for forever either.

The silver lining here is that being in need develops the gift of empathy. There will come a time in the future when you'll be willing and eager to repay the kindnesses you receive. You will recognize and understand the needs of others when you see them and will offer assistance if you can. It may be years later. The circumstances and the people involved may be very different, but you will still be anxious to help if you can.

Recognize that it's not your fault that you have limitations now. Try to remember that nothing stays the same. Live your life the best that you can, and make the most of every moment, even if many of them are spent on the couch.

Discussion Questions:

> *If you've been pregnant while having FM symptoms describe your experience.*
> *How did you deal with it?*
> *Did you experience postpartum depression? What was that like?*

Chapter 7

Yes, it Hurts!

I never knew what pain was until I had my first bout with a pinched nerve in my spine. It was diagnosed incorrectly for thirty-five years. Until about ten years ago, it was thought to be a muscular condition. As such, I was prescribed moist heat, anti-inflammatories, muscle relaxants and a very mild opiate. None of it worked. The best I could hope for was enough medication to put me to sleep until the episode subsided on its own.

When the pain worsened to the point where each jolt was severe enough to move my body involuntarily, one doctor bravely labeled it "zoster sine herpete," the technical name for shingles with no rash, a condition other doctors have told me doesn't exist. Post-herpetic neuralgia, a highly painful chronic condition that can result from having had shingles while in an immune-suppressed state, is only slightly more commonly known. That diagnosis was bandied around as well.

Strangely, for a condition about which so little is known and whose very existence is in question, I happen to know several people who have had such a diagnosis (shingles without rash) and many more who have had the symptoms. Not all of them have FM.

For many years, each episode of my condition responded to the combination of an anti-viral drug and Codeine. I would take them both, sleep for a few hours, and awaken pain free. Unfortunately, in time that treatment became ineffective. In retrospect, it was likely that only the Codeine had any effect. I suspect that a higher dose might have lessened my pain. Instead, a different opiate was prescribed. It provided relief initially, but also became ineffective with time.

As the years went on, the episodes became more frequent and lasted longer. When the pain became unbearable, I'd go to the Emergency Room. There I'd be given an injection of some stronger pain reliever, and the pain would be gone. Often, however, the pain would reappear several hours after leaving the hospital and returning home.

The pain was (and continues to be) always in exactly the same spot, just under my left shoulder blade near my spine. Because I've had different health insurance plans over the years, I've also had different doctors and a wide range of diagnoses.

One neurologist I saw was convinced I had RSD (reflex sympathetic dystrophy), a rare disorder of the sympathetic nervous system. For this I was given Botox injections into the problem muscle every 3 months. It made little difference in the frequency or severity of my pain. Actually, the injection itself inevitably caused a major pain episode the following day. I decided it was more hurtful than helpful.

I've also been referred to pain management specialists where I was given various spinal injections. Not only were they totally ineffective, each injection brought on an even worse pain episode the next day.

I was also prescribed trigger point injections with a combination of Marcaine and Cortisone. Depending upon who did it and whether or not I was having symptoms at the time of the injection, they produced varying degrees of relief. Most recently, due to the spread of acute pain to my rib cage, I have received yet another diagnosis. My doctors now agree that there's a pinched nerve in my spinal column. A very small dose of Pamelor worked miraculously well for the first 5 days to quiet that nerve, at which point the side effects of the drug became more severe than the symptoms.

It was a chiropractor who initially provided some of the best relief I've had. It became apparent that my pain episodes occurred whenever my spine was crooked. If my spine was adjusted when I first became aware of discomfort in the area, the pain could be prevented. He also prescribed a series of strengthening exercises for the muscles around my spine to help keep it straight. The frequency of my pain lessened significantly. I've learned to recognize when my back is crooked, and I get myself adjusted as quickly as possible.

Even more recently, I've been seeing a physiatrist (a physical medicine doctor). His explanation for my long-term acute pain is myofascial pain syndrome. Of all the diagnoses I've received over the years, this one makes the most sense to me. It is also commonly associated with fibromyalgia. Unfortunately there is no cure and little that can be done to address the pain. I have, however, been referred to a physical therapist who has been quite helpful – especially now that my severe pain has expanded to include the back of my head in addition to my upper back.

My new pain has been labeled occipital neuralgia by my physiatrist. It, too, is the result of myofascial pain syndrome. It is even initiated by the same trigger point. When the muscles of my shoulders and neck tighten up (as they do when I spend more time than I should working at my computer without taking a break) that muscle tightness compresses the nerve and starts the pain. Once the nerve is irritated, it has to get worse before it gets better. Only exercise (which itself is painful) can relax the muscles. Some people are fortunate to be able to tolerate medications like muscle relaxants and anti-inflammatories that help to relieve the pressure on the muscles. I'm not one of them.

My alternative is physical therapy. I now have exercises that are effective for relieving the head pain after about 2 weeks of doing them religiously at least 3 times a day. I've also purchased a foam roller which I place on the floor, then roll back and forth on top of it. I hear the same cracking noises I heard when having chiropractic adjustments. The results appear to be the same. It's also more convenient and far less expensive. In addition, I continue to do strengthening exercises every day. My entire focus is on prevention. Once the pain begins I cease to function There is little I can do besides take opiate drugs. Although I'm very grateful for their effectiveness, I'm frightened to think of the long-term effects on my internal organs and the tolerance I'm building up. Already, I need twice the amount I was initially prescribed 8 years ago. I certainly wish the medical community would come up with some safer but equally effective pain relievers!

I was fortunate to have been referred to Kaiser's pain management program. It was conducted by three wonderful professionals: an M.D. (who is a pain specialist), a psychologist and a physical therapist. The program is intense. It requires attending two 3-hr. sessions per week for six weeks as well as doing lots of reading and homework.

After the initial evaluation and pain reduction using medication, the 6 week learning program begins. The goal of the program is to give patients the tools to tolerate/lessen their pain without the use of medication. I will forever be grateful for that experience. Their persistent pain management doctor (working in conjunction with an allergist for my severe side effects) finally prescribed an opiate strong enough to completely control the acute pain from my pinched nerve episodes and prevented my frequent Emergency Room visits. I have some slight side effects from the drug, but they're not nearly as severe as the pain is. And after an allergist confirmed they are indeed side effects I experience rather than an allergy, I'm not frightened to take the medication when I need it. I wonder what they're doing in the ER with all their free time without me these days?

What I've been describing is acute pain. It is defined as having an identifiable source and is brief in duration. Of course, "brief" is relative and doesn't feel so brief if you're the one who's experiencing it. And if acute pain occurs over and over again it becomes labeled as chronic.

Fibromyalgia, on the other hand, is truly chronic pain. This is pain that does not go away with time. Fortunately, it is not life-threatening, although it can really make life miserable. One of the most challenging aspects of chronic pain is convincing another person (sometimes even your doctor) that your pain is real.

A factor that contributes to the difficulty is that people with fibromyalgia rarely look sick. People constantly say to me, "But you look really healthy!" The next person may live to regret those words.!! What I want to tell each one of them is to try being me for a week. Instead, I usually just smile and say "thank you."

The truth of the matter is that FM pain gnaws and burns and aches and grates its way into your life. Hour after hour, day after day, it's enough to drive you to despair. The emotional roller coaster ride just adds to the pain. On the occasional good day you begin to get hopeful about the future. You make plans to do things you enjoy. Then the barometric pressure changes or something stressful happens or you get overly enthusiastic and overdo it, and suddenly your good day is only a memory. So, how do you deal with it?

If you're fortunate enough to have a pain management program such as Kaiser's at your disposal, I highly recommend it. I learned enough about controlling pain without the use of medication there that I could write an entire book on that topic.

If there's no such program available to you, here are some things that have been helpful to me:

- Employ breathing techniques. These can be so powerful that I've devoted an entire chapter to them. (See "Take a Deep Breath")
- Distract yourself. Find something that you can really focus on. It might be music – anything from Mozart to Eminem – whatever pleases you. Or sing. Or dance (even if only while sitting in a chair). Paint a picture. Have a sexual encounter. Do anything that makes you happy.
- Employ one of the Touch Therapies (See Chapter with that title)
- Call a friend on the phone and talk about anything other than your pain.
- Meditate or pray or both – whatever works for you. (See Chapter 16)
- Deep relaxation
- Try medical marijuana – but only if it's legal in your state and you have a recommendation to use it. Look for a strain that is high in CBD (cannabidiol) which is the pain-relieving content of the plant. Start with a tiny amount. For myself, I nearly gave up when the dose prescribed on the bottle didn't alleviate my pain. However, when I

increased the dose I received the promised result. Always keep in mind that fibromyalgia patients are known to have unique reactions to ingested substances. Cannabis is no exception.

- Learn to use a TENS unit. Have a physical therapist instruct you in the correct placement for your specific pain.
- Watch a funny movie. Keep a constant supply available of things that make you laugh. Bring them out whenever you're in pain. Laughter and sex produce the same pain-fighting endorphins as morphine does.
- Take a hot bath. Add some Epsom Salts if you have them. The magnesium they contain will relax your muscles and thereby reduce pain. (Do be aware that if you're extremely sensitive to magnesium – as I am – diarrhea might be the result)
- Gentle rubs with capsaicin creams are sometimes effective. They bring increased heat and blood flow to painful areas, which is a good thing. But, be very careful if you have sensitive skin like mine. Capsaicin is made from hot red peppers. It's very strong, and it may burn you.
- Try Salonpas patches, Tiger Balm or Biofreeze on your most painful places.
- Have an acupuncture treatment.
- Use heat or ice or alternate between the two. (every 5 minutes or so). You can make your own ice pack by freezing 3 cups of water along with 1 cup of isopropyl alcohol in a plastic zip lock bag placed inside a second zip lock bag. If it's too slushy, add water. If it's too solid, add more alcohol.
- Learn visualization techniques or participate in Guided Imagery. YouTube is a good source for this.

- Try hypnotherapy. I've used a free App found on Amazon called Fast Healing: Power of the Mind by Rachael Meddows. It takes only 35 minutes, and I have found it to be very helpful.
- Try biofeedback.
- Do regular stretching and exercise.
- Learn and use the Tapping Solution (www.thetappingsolution.com) also known as EFT (Emotional Freedom Technique)
- Do Laughter Yoga.

The basis for many of the above techniques is that the mind and the body are connected. If you can focus the mind on something other than pain, your pain will subside. It can only handle one function at a time. If you're having an acute episode, these techniques may not alleviate your pain entirely, but they can help get you through until your medication takes effect or your extreme discomfort subsides.

Never forget how powerful the mind is. If you're doubtful, think about the placebo effect or psychosomatic illnesses. Know that the more you practice the above techniques, the better they will work for you.

I also use a psychological technique as a means of tolerating my pain. I categorize it as either "good" or "bad. "Good" pain is the result of having enjoyed myself too much - either standing too long or walking too far in some pleasurable pursuit. The next day, when the aching begins, I just remind myself of the fun I had, and the pain becomes easier to bear.

"Bad" pain is more difficult to tolerate. It can often be attributed to poor sleep, over-activity, repetitive motion, or weather changes. Sometimes it's caused by nothing at all. It is definitely not the result of enjoyment. It has no redeeming value. This pain challenges all of my coping skills.

Hypnotherapy done by a licensed psychologist is another option to consider. My experience with seeing a hypnotherapist was nothing like I expected it would be. Instead of dangling a shiny object in front of my eyes to focus on and suggesting that, "You feel sleepy", she invited me to get comfortable on her recliner. She interviewed me for about half an hour to learn what was happening in my life that might be preventing me from sleeping – the problem I was there to address. She then asked me to put my cell phone in a recording mode and to lie back and close my eyes. In a very soothing voice she gave some instructions for relaxation that put me to sleep quite quickly. I left with that recording, played it every night for a week or so, and haven't had a problem sleeping since then. Whether my inability to fall asleep was cured by hypnosis or whether it was a problem that was about to cure itself anyway is anybody's guess. I prefer to think my very expensive session with the hypnotherapist was worth the money I spent.

I've learned it's easier to prevent pain than it is to heal it. Done regularly, stretching prevents many of the knots and spasms responsible for much of FM pain. In my view, there's no better stretching program than Qi Gong. Read a book, take a class, watch Youtube videos, but learn to do it and do it daily. It only takes a few minutes, and the positive effects on your body and your mind can be truly life changing.

If none of these non-medication techniques is successful in managing your pain, consider asking your doctor to try one of the 3 prescription drugs now available for treatment of FM. As a last resort, try a narcotic. Numerous studies have demonstrated that people who use opiates for short-term relief of severe pain DO NOT get addicted to opiates. In a 1982 article in Pain magazine, a survey of physicians and nurses who treated more than 10,000 patients (all on opiates) in 93 burn units for highly-painful debridement procedures reported only 12% of patients developed addiction after leaving the hospital. Of these, all but one reported a history of prior substance abuse.

Several years ago I took Vicodin three times a day for several months because of unrelenting pain in my head, neck, shoulders, hips and knees. I couldn't have functioned without it. Because I truly needed it, I didn't feel drugged, and I didn't become addicted. I was able to get up and go to work and perform my job effectively. As my pain subsided, I only took the pill at night to help me sleep. As time went on, I needed less and less until eventually I needed none at all. I suffered no withdrawal symptoms and at no time did I desire to take more than was prescribed.

Today the country is facing an opioid crisis. However, many pain specialists agree that the problem is with street drugs rather than prescription drugs. In many instances, the overdoses in question happen by accident – often the result of mixing an opiate with a benzodiazepine class of drugs – and often with the elderly whose bodies process medications differently than they once did. Don't be discouraged. If nothing else relieves your pain ask for help.

My point is: Narcotics can help you through the bad times. Unless you happen to have a highly addictive gene (and you're probably already aware of it if you do) your body will tell you when you don't need the drug any more. As you already know, flares don't last forever. You will feel better eventually. But there's no need to be miserable while you wait.

Discussion Questions:

> *What is the first thing you do when your pain worsens?*
> *What is the most effective non-pharmaceutical technique you employ?*
> *Have you had success with one of the new fibromyalgia medications?*
> *Which symptoms have improved?*

Chapter 8

Fibrofog or
Who moved my bookmark?

Of all the fibromyalgia symptoms I know, cognitive difficulties are the most difficult to describe. Basically, there are two types. The first is a lack of short term memory. That one is quite common in the elderly population as well as in FM. The second type is often referred to as "fibrofog". Between the two, they are probably responsible for more FM disability filings than any other symptom. They were definitely the cause of mine.

Here's an example of what can happen with your memory: You meet your boss in the hallway where you have neither paper nor pen with which to write. He rattles off three things he needs you to accomplish before the end of the day. You nod, desperately repeating these words in your head over and over, trying not to be rude by ignoring the rest of what he's saying. By the time you get back to your desk, you can remember the last task and part of the second task. The first one has completely vanished from your mind.

This development can be devastating to a person like me who took pride in her memory from her earliest years. At one time I accurately remembered nearly everything I read or heard: names, numbers, dates, facts, anything and everything. In school I was teased about the obscure things I could call to mind after having read them only once in the newspaper or a magazine article. In textbooks I could remember the exact location on the page where I had seen a particular word or fact. That all changed with FM.

As my FM symptoms worsened, my mind became more muddled (even without pain medication). My corporate finance job became a daily struggle. Even routine tasks I could previously perform without blinking became impossible. I couldn't add the same column of numbers twice and get the same answer. Not appearing as confused as I felt was a major accomplishment each day.

You can work in pain (unless it's acute). You can work without sleep (unless it's chronic). You can work with Irritable Bowel Syndrome (if the rest room isn't too far from your workplace). You can deal with all of the other FM symptoms as well, although it's no walk in the park. But there's no way you can maintain a responsible job if you suffer from fibrofog. I know. Eventually the stress of living this way resulted in my filing for disability. By that time my brain felt like a wad of cotton candy and functioned about as well.

How I envy people who can remember the details of books they've read and the movies they've seen. I cannot. If I'm lucky, I can remember the beginning until I get to the end. Some days even that is more than I can do. Have you ever picked up a book you started to read several days before, looked at the bookmarked page and not recognized a single thing on it? Not a name, not a place, who was doing what to whom? So you back up a page or two to look for clues. Still nothing. Back up a few more pages, then a few more. When you finally put the book down after reading for half an hour you wind up putting the bookmark in a place more toward the beginning of the book than you were when you started reading? That's what it's like to have fibrofog. It can be very discouraging for those of us who really want to keep up with the world or who want to learn something new. So, what can be done about it? Here are a few suggestions:

If you're trying to absorb new material, try playing some Mozart while you're reading or listening to educational material. Don't listen to anything else. Other music is more distracting than helpful. Scientists at Stanford University revealed the molecular basis for what is now known as the Mozart Effect. I don't pretend to understand it, but I know it has something to do with the rhythm. The steady beat of music at a very particular speed actually breaks up the music into pieces the brain can store (along with the new information you're reading) into a place where it can be recalled when it's needed. It sounds a bit bizarre, but it does work.

If you don't own any of Mozart's music, go to your public library and borrow some. They're certain to have it available in any format you need. In particular, look for his piano sonatas. Using this technique has an unexpected bonus. In a short time you'll learn to appreciate and even to recognize Mozart compositions when you hear them. You'll be pleasantly surprised by how impressed people will be when you do.

In addition to helping with fibrofog, studies done at the University of Granada found that listening to music once a day over a 4-week time period reduced pain and depression symptoms. The theory is that by stimulating the brain with pleasant sounds, you drown out the unpleasant feelings.

We've always known that a good way to learn something is to teach it to somebody else. So plan to tell someone about what you're reading. Knowing you're going to do this helps you to summarize in your mind what you've just read. This technique works well for movies, too, but only if it's done shortly after you've seen it. If you wait even a day or two, it may be too late.

Console yourself with the fact that even if you can't remember a single thing about a movie you've seen or a book you've read a day or a week before, it wasn't a waste of time. You enjoyed it at the time. Learn to be grateful for that. Some time in the future you'll be able to enjoy it again as if it were totally new!

My final suggestion is to read or listen to something you'd like to learn for only very short intervals. This isn't as crazy as it sounds either. Studies done by Dr. Mihaly Czikszentmihalyi, a well-known educator and former head of the Psychology Department at the University of Chicago, showed that people most often remember the first thing and the last thing they read. So, the trick is not to have too much in the middle to forget. So, read a couple of pages, then file a couple of fingernails. Read a few more pages, then file a couple more. Read a little more, and go get a glass of water. Get the idea?

Keep in mind that cognitive difficulties, like most FM symptoms, are much more severe when you're tired. If there's something you really want to read or create or to learn, do it when you feel as rested as possible. For me, I function best between 11 a.m. and 2 p.m. Then I begin to go downhill. By 4:30 I need at least an hour's nap to get through dinnertime and the early evening. Then I get revived about 10:00 p.m. This is both a good and a bad thing. It's good in that I feel creative at that time; it's bad in that if I begin to read or to write, I get in the flow and I'm liable to be up most of the night. Lack of sleep results in increased pain the next day, and I have no one to blame but myself. The lesson to be learned here is to know what works best for you and to act accordingly.

Above all, don't despair. Any goal is reachable when you have fibromyalgia. It may take a little longer or you may need to follow an uncharted route. But you can get there. Look at me. My goal was to write a book to help others deal with FM. Yes, it took me at least twice as long as it would have taken someone else, but with patience and perseverance, I did it. Twice!

Don't let FM stop you from reaching your goals. Whatever it is you want to do, it's possible. You just need to find the tools that work for you and use them.

Discussion Questions:

> *When do you experience your worst cognitive problems?*
> *What techniques have you used successfully to improve your memory?*
> *What memory aides have you purchased that were worth the price?*

Chapter 9

Irritable Everything

A wicked ruler named Irritable Bowel Syndrome (IBS) governs my life. It has caused me to miss good times and bad, both social and professional. Over the years my non-attendance at various places has been interpreted as a social snub by some, as an insult by others, and often as a statement I never intended to make. In most cases, I didn't feel obligated to explain my bodily malfunction to the injured party. Mostly, I just allowed people to believe what they wanted. That may have diminished my social circle, but it kept my dignity intact. I've been viewed as a bit of snob my entire life when the real problem was an irritable bowel accompanied by abdominal pain and profound fatigue.

During my working life, only one of my bosses ever understood fibromyalgia and the myriad symptoms it causes. The others made it clear to all employees (while looking directly at me) that their personal problems should remain at home. I never attempted to explain my life to them. Rather I just tried harder when I was there to make up for the frequent times when I wasn't. Hello, stress!

Does this scenario sound familiar? I'm busy getting ready for work. There's an important meeting that day, so I decide to wear the new suit I bought earlier in the week. I assemble my best accessories, spend extra time with my hair and make-up, arrange the files I'd studied the night before so I might answer questions intelligently even in the midst of fibrofog.

Time to get dressed. What's wrong? The skirt that fit like a glove when I bought it 3 days ago refuses to button at my waist. The zipper won't go all the way up. There's no way I can wear it. Looking in the mirror, I see the reason why. IBS bloat has struck again!

I'm running out of time, starting to feel frantic. I rummage through the closet to locate something else that matches the accessories now lined up on my bed. Can't find anything! I tell myself to relax. Surely there's something that will stretch over my extended belly.

Alas, one dress fits but it doesn't match the accessories. So, back to the closet I go in search of different shoes, a belt that matches, silver rather than gold jewelry. I can't find the mate to the hoop in my ear. A glance at the clock says my car should have pulled out of the driveway three minutes ago to avoid the traffic crunch. And then I start to feel crampy.

"Not now," I pray, loitering another 5 minutes close to the bathroom, wondering if I can accomplish the fifteen-minute drive to work without an accident. (I'm not talking about a traffic accident here, although that, too, would be a distinct possibility.) I watch the second hand on the clock tick slowly around.

No choice. I must leave. Another 5 minutes and the freeway traffic will make me an hour late for the meeting with my out-of-town clients - a meeting that I, myself, scheduled. Time's up! I run to the car and pray for the best, clenching my muscles all the way and praying the Imodium will work by the time I reach my destination.

This is not an unusual day for someone with IBS. It causes havoc in the workplace as well as in our social lives. It's what makes a lot of us shun social engagements and avoid making new friends who require new explanations. Dating? Forget it!

However, your IBS may be very different from mine. If it's precipitated by a particular food or drink, you may successfully control it by just abstaining from those things. Keeping a food journal for a couple of weeks can help you identify the culprit(s). Or perhaps one of the medications now available will control it for you. Or your symptoms may occur so seldom that it's really not that big of a problem for you.

Mine wasn't so easy to control. After testing for conventional food allergies proved negative except for a mild lactose intolerance and an allergy to pineapple, I proceeded to an alternative practitioner who tested me for food sensitivities. That's where I learned that wheat and soy were my worst enemies. After removing them completely from my diet and showing only slight improvement, I removed raw vegetables from my diet in favor of only cooked ones which are easier to digest. Next I eliminated red meat. My problem remains ongoing, but the results of straying from my current dietary restrictions are easily recognizable. My inability to tolerate any of the drugs available to treat IBS has been an unfortunate situation for me as well. So, I continue to struggle.

There are many variations of IBS. In addition to IBS-D (with diarrhea) there is IBS-C (meaning with constipation). There is also a combination of both. Yet another category of patients have only pain with neither diarrhea nor constipation.

Your irritable bladder may be more bothersome for you than your IBS is. Having been plagued with both of them more times than I care to remember, I find it much easier to live with an irritable bladder than it is to live with IBS. I've recently learned there can be more than frequency and urgency involved. Some people experience pain similar to that which is typical of a urinary tract infection (UTI) even though no bacteria is involved. It can be caused by excess acidity in the urine. Certain foods (known as bladder irritants) can be the cause. I now keep a list and make certain I haven't overindulged in any of them before I request a urinalysis for a suspected urinary tract infection.

If incontinence is your issue, there are some helpful programs conducted by physical therapists. The one I attended had 40 people in it – about half women, half men. To learn if there's such a program in your area, call a local urologist's office or ask your GP.

The class I attended taught techniques for relaxing the bladder and increasing the amount it will hold before feeling the urge. We also learned exercises to strengthen the sphincter muscles, and had a tutorial on which foods (mainly citrus and sugar) are bladder irritants. Keeping a diary of which liquids and what quantity of liquid is drunk each day will help to identify and eliminate your triggers.

I also learned that a lot of what we do is habit. Using the bathroom before we leave the house, no matter where we're going, even if we just went 15 minutes before, is just a habit. Did you know that the normal interval between urination is 3-4 hours? After comparing it to the half hour or so that was more normal for me I was sufficiently motivated to follow up on what I'd learned. It took a little time and practice, but I'm much better now than I was before.

Knowing the location of rest rooms is essential if you're bothered by either irritable bladder or IBS. I have the layouts of most grocery store chains in Southern California emblazoned on my brain. There's a particular grocery store chain near my home that recently underwent a total remodel of all their stores. Their bright new bathrooms are located adjacent to the front door. I always buy an item or two out of gratitude when I run in to use one of them.

Londoners have the right idea. "Loos" (their equivalent of our porta-potties but cleaner) are located like phone booths on every street corner. Unfortunately, the rainy weather there plays havoc with my disposition and increases my muscle pain. I guess there are trade-offs for everything – no matter where you choose to live.

Airplane travel is a real challenge if you suffer from one of these two "irritables". With all those people on the plane and only one or possibly two facilities located front and back, what do you do if you need to use one in a big hurry? Newer security regulations even prevent you from lining up to be next. You must remain in your seat until the "vacant" sign is visible. The stress of this situation can be overwhelming. The sad result is that I visit my grandchild a lot less frequently than I would like to.

Long car trips can be even more of a challenge, especially if you haven't driven the route before. You can pretty much assume a fast food outlet will be located at a freeway exit, but not always. I have a cupboard full of paper maps on which I've drawn little red circles on the places where there's an easily accessible restroom at the exit - like a McDonald's or a Burger King or a gas station where you don't have to stand in line to get a key. I'm thinking of selling my maps to AAA. There's probably a phone app that will tell the location of all fast food outlets along a given route. However, my iPhone skills have yet to take me that far.

Technology has come a long way toward developing products that are helpful for people with "irritable" issues. There are protective products available today that can really help if you're unsure where the next bathroom will be located. Whether you choose to use them "Depends" on how severe your problem is and how desperate you feel.

This is one area in which men have a definite advantage. On a long car trip, for example, they can always carry a large empty jar in the backseat, just in case. Only recently has there been a similar product developed for women. It's called a "She-wee" or a female urinal. Although it's not really easy to use, I suppose it could be a godsend if you're stuck in traffic or if there's no freeway exit in sight.

It's more socially acceptable to admit to having an irritable bladder than to having irritable bowel syndrome. Always needing to "pee" can even be viewed as a cute, feminine peccadillo. In contrast, there's nothing the least bit charming about the horrible gas pains, diarrhea, nausea and other embarrassing symptoms that accompany IBS-D.

Just like other fibromyalgia symptoms, IBS and irritable bladder are not permanent afflictions. Episodes will come and go. There will be good times and bad. With time and patience, you will learn what triggers an attack for you, and you will change your life accordingly. Hopefully, these symptoms won't occur in conjunction with other problems and won't require the drastic changes I found it necessary to make, like eliminating wheat, dairy and raw vegetables from my diet. But, if that should happen, so be it.

As in every area of life, attitude is everything. If you can learn to embrace change, to think of it as an adventure, as something positive, very good things can result. Look at me! Here I am clear across the country, living in sunny, Southern California, in a house near the ocean, with a wonderful new husband, an adorable little dog, and a one-hour flight away from my first grandchild. I would have missed all these things had I continued to endure my miserable existence in upstate New York (no offense, New Yorkers).

Discussion Questions:

> *What techniques do you use to prevent episodes of IBS or irritable bladder?*
> *What situations or foods trigger episodes for you?*

Chapter 10

What's That Smell?

It's nearly as difficult to explain Multiple Chemical Sensitivity (MCS) to someone who doesn't have it, as it is to explain fibromyalgia. It's hard to believe that an odor could cause symptoms like headache, nausea, fatigue, confusion and body pain, especially when that odor isn't unpleasant to most people, and it's completely undetectable by others.

A co-worker once brought me a beautiful bouquet of pink peonies from his garden. Their perfume was so strong I had to leave work by mid-morning. At home, I lay on the couch, bleary-eyed, nauseous and headachy for the next 2 days. I didn't dare tell the people at work why I was home. For sure they would have thought I was crazy. Even I began to wonder about my sanity. But those peonies were definitely responsible. I could taste their scent.

My husband recently planted an elegant rose garden below my bedroom window. Although I was afraid of sounding ungrateful, I had to insist the design be rearranged, locating the scented bushes as far away from the house as possible. Although roses are my favorite flower to look it, their smell is definitely a problem for me.

Not all plants are problematic. Some can be helpful

for sensitive people like me. The following list indicates plants that are reported to reduce the air concentration of the three most common indoor scented pollutants.

Formaldehyde

Sources: foam insulation, plywood, clothes, carpeting, furniture, paper goods, household cleaners.
Suitable plants: Philodendron, spider plant, golden pothos, chrysanthemum, Sanseveria (snake plant).

Benzene

Sources: tobacco smoke, petrol, synthetic fibers, plastics, inks, oils, detergents, rubber.
Suitable plants: English Ivy, Dracaena marginata, chrysanthemum, gerbera, peace lily.

Trichloroethylene

Sources: Dry cleaning fluid, inks, paints, varnishes, lacquers, adhesives.
Suitable plants: Gerbera, chrysanthemum, peace lily, dracaena marginata.

Another potential problem on the homefront is your mattress. I purchased a new one two years ago, and received an unwelcome education. The smell was noticeable as they were unwrapping the product in my bedroom, and I said so. I then called the salesman who assured me it was only because the item had been stored in plastic. Hours later the smell hadn't dissipated one bit. At that point, my husband and I dragged both the mattress and box spring out to the patio where it remained until bedtime. It smelled a bit better so we dragged it back inside. Exhausted from all the physical effort, I quickly fell asleep on it. Two hours later I awoke with a severe headache, feeling nauseous. I slept on the couch the rest of the night. The next day we dragged the mattress outside again. I tried to sleep on it one more night, this time developing a rash on my legs along with burning eyes, nausea and a sickening chemical taste. By now the smell had permeated the entire house. We wrapped the mattress in aluminum foil and plastic and dragged it outside one last time.

Resolving the issue was another dilemma. The store refused to take it back, saying it was illegal to return mattresses. I then contacted the Serta area representative. After hearing my tale of woe, he authorized a full refund to the store. After two weeks they agreed to pick it up for a $100 fee. Meanwhile I studied everything I should have known before I made that purchase. This is what I learned.

There are regulations governing flame retardancy for mattresses that differ from state to state. The original intent was commendable. It was to save lives. But the result is a disaster for a lot of people. As you can imagine, the cheapest product available to make a mattress flame retardant is most widely used. That product is boric acid – yes, the same thing used to kill cockroaches. The Agency for Toxic Substances and Disease Registry (ATSDR) a division of the Center for Disease Control (CDC) cites Boron/Boric Acid as one of 275 substances "which pose the most significant potential threat to human health". If you rub a piece of black paper on top of your box spring chances are you'll see white powder. That's the culprit.

But take heart: I also learned there are organic mattresses on the market that are naturally fireproof. They need no chemical fire retardants added to them.

Although pricey, I knew that one of them needed to be my choice. I tested each variety available by lying on them in the store (to which I brought my pillow). After testing the cotton ones and the wool ones I finally decided on an organic latex one made by Savvy Rest. I'm delighted with my purchase.

Over the years I've learned how to avoid most of the fumes that make me sick, although I've yet to figure out how to buy unscented soap without spending time in the scented soap aisle of the grocery store. It's impossible to push a cart with one hand while holding your nose with the other. So, trips to the market often result in headaches and increased pain and fatigue. My new plan is to occasionally splurge and pay the money to have my groceries delivered. That's when I'll purchase all my cleaning products in order to avoid the smells in the store.

Any public place is a potential hazard for someone with MCS. I've had to change seats in movie theaters and change tables in restaurants because of someone's perfume or aftershave. I can only get my hair cut first thing in the morning - before the fumes from all the products they use build up in the shop.

I give credit to department stores. They've become sensitive to the issue. Now they ask before spritzing you with perfume the way they used to do.

Once, when I was still a working lady, floor tile was being installed in the office downstairs from mine. Shortly after they opened the can of glue, I could taste the fumes and became nauseous. That smell drove me out of the building and kept me home for nearly a week.

After that, I planned my vacations whenever nearby offices were being renovated. If I had no vacation days left, I called in sick. It was easier to stay at home than to explain my sudden departure. Other people commented on smells from time to time, but they just kept on working. I hated myself for being such a wimp. I'd never heard of MCS at the time.

I was nauseous for several weeks after having our home tented for termites several years ago. Nearly four years later I could still conjure up the smell. What would it have been like if we'd not opted for the extra-cost, so-called "odorless" spray? Last year our house needed tenting again. I was really concerned, trying to figure out where I could live until the smell dissipated. I shouldn't have worried. In the past few years a different chemical is being used – at least in California. Now, when they say odorless, they really mean it. When we returned home after a 2-day tenting, there was no odor apparent to me at all. What a relief! Now, if they'd only find a way to do the process that didn't involve emptying all the food out of the house or double-bagging anything that was left. That was one huge effort – one I don't wish to undertake again any time soon.

The fact is that people with FM are overly sensitive to many things, including smells. There is even a school of thought that says overexposure to chemicals and its resultant autoimmune response may be the total cause of fibromyalgia. This same response is thought to be responsible for Gulf War Syndrome. Its symptoms are very similar to those of FM (i.e. total body pain, fatigue, cognitive difficulties and sleep problems).

I'm not pleased that our soldiers have experienced FM symptoms, but because of the prevalence of Gulf War Syndrome, the Department of Defense has allocated an increase in the previously minimal funding allocated to the National Institute of Health (NIH) to study our common disorder. Helping our veterans may also help us.

Until a cure for fibromyalgia is found, be aware that intense odors may exacerbate its symptoms. Try to avoid places where you're likely to have problems. Breathe as much outside air as possible. Always sleep with a window open, and advise friends and family members that their grooming products may cause you problems.

I'm pleased to note that many group meetings are now being declared no-scent zones. I sing with a Sweet Adelines group that is very serious about their scent-free policy. Apparently, even people without fibromyalgia can be affected by strong odors.

Speak out in favor of organic foods and chemical-free products. Support companies that produce healthy products whenever you can. I know that sometimes organic foods are way out of the average person's budget, but if there's only a small difference in price, try to choose organic.

Watch for legislation that supports healthy living and contact your government representative's office to voice your support. This is an area where being pro-active can really make a difference.

Discussion Questions:

> *What triggers an MCS episode for you? What symptoms does it cause?*
> *How do you avoid MCS episodes?*
> *How do you describe MCS to others who are not affected?*

Chapter 11

To Sleep perchance to Dream!

O.K. I'll settle for sleeping, although a non drug-induced dream once in a while would be a lovely bonus. Sleep problems are so common to fibromyalgia that some specialists believe it's the actual cause rather than just a symptom. Everyone agrees that sleep issues increase pain and fatigue. As apnea is the most common of these issues, I agreed to a sleep study to rule it out.

Apnea stops your breathing long enough for the lungs to signal your brain that they need more air. The brain then lifts you out of deep sleep so you can take a breath. With apnea, this happens so frequently that you get very little deep sleep and awaken feeling as tired as when you went to bed. Although it sounds trivial, the condition can be deadly.

The good news is that there are machines that can help. Called CPAP's (short for Continuous Positive Airway Pressure), they supply a constant flow of oxygen to the lungs so that awakening to breathe becomes unnecessary. They are available only by prescription and only after apnea has been confirmed. When my first study was done in 2001 a machine cost $2,500.

A call to my insurance company confirmed they would pay for the study, and they referred me to a local firm that specialized in performing these tests. The location of the study should have been a clue that this organization might be less than professional. But I reasoned that because people slept at motels, it was a logical place to conduct a sleep study. Moreover, my insurance company recommended this organization, so they must be legitimate.

As instructed I arrived at Room #201 at 10 p.m. carrying my little overnight bag. A huge bearded man with a foreign accent ushered me into the harshly lit living area of the motel suite. He invited me to sit at the dining table across from some technical apparatus with a large-screen monitor and gave me a stack of paperwork to complete. As I outlined my past history in great detail I waited for the professional - perhaps a doctor or at least a female - to arrive. None did. It was to be just this big brute and me.

After finishing the paperwork, my instructions were to step into the adjoining bedroom and change into my nightclothes. After that, I was to return to the table where wires would be attached to my body. These wires would attach to the machine next to the bed where I would sleep. The "brute" in the dining area would spend the night monitoring the machines' activity while I slept.

Slept???? Was he kidding? I don't sleep in strange beds even under the very best of conditions! Ambien goes with me wherever I travel. But no drugs were allowed (I was told) as they would likely skew the test results.

Even before the lights went out, I knew there was little chance of sleep; but I was desperate for help. I hadn't felt rested in months, and my pain was worsening as a result. So, I decided I'd try to forget about the man lurking in the next room and do the best I could. With any luck my current state of sleep deprivation was severe enough that I might manage an hour or two.

I lay there in the darkness, wires connected to every limb, and a contraption wrapped around my forehead that resembled the headgear on Frankenstein's monster. I jumped at every sound while employing every sleep-inducing technique I'd ever learned. And there were many!

Concentrating on relaxing one muscle at a time, my body instead became stiff as a board. Taking a mental vacation to my favorite place had no effect. Recalling the names of the streets I'd passed on my long walk to high school (a technique I'd successfully used in the past) didn't work either. I tried counting blessings (instead of sheep). But the harder I tried to sleep, the more awake I became. It was an effort just to keep my eyes closed.

And then the commotion began. First, loud footsteps, then a giggling female voice, followed by a masculine snort. With the bed positioned next to the window and the equipment on the opposite side, sitting up and parting the blackout drapes so I could peak outside was my next move. An open metal staircase was close enough to touch. All I saw were two feet clad in backless, high-heeled, wooden-soled shoes clanging loudly on every step. Then two people collapsed in a heap in front of me, laughing loudly and shushing each other. Eventually they clomped noisily via the outside corridor to a distant room and banged the door shut.

I was determined not to let that interruption ruin my chance for a CPAP machine. Once again I employed my sleep-inducing techniques. This time I imagined I was on my way to my childhood school. Somewhere between Oswego Street and Lincoln Avenue a door slammed again. Then I heard more footsteps, quieter this time, but banging just as loudly down the stairs and retreating into the distance.

I said to myself. "Now that that's over, I can finally go to sleep." And I did try. I slipped back into my "vacation" mode again. This time it worked quite well. There I was, sailing blissfully across the lake in a gentle breeze on a warm sunny day. I was almost asleep.

Then came the familiar female voice in the distance, the same clomping footsteps. This time there was no conversation, but definitely 2 peoples' footsteps stomping up the stairs. Another door banging shut. And so it went - every 30 minutes or so, all night long. Up the stairs, down the stairs, over and over. It took a while for my naive little self to realize what was going on. The woman wearing the wooden clogs was conducting a "night time business"!

Periodically, the "gorilla" in the next room would poke his head in the door to ask if I was all right or to adjust a wire or two. I told him about the noise, but he assured me I only needed to sleep a couple of hours for him to get the results he needed. He encouraged me to try harder.

As the night wore on, the usual pain in my muscles and joints increased to such a state that I was fighting back tears at 5 a.m. when my torturer decided to call it quits. I'd only managed to doze lightly for about 35 minutes, not nearly enough time to produce any significant data. Totally frustrated, I got dressed and went home.

I'd suffered through a thoroughly miserable night for absolutely no purpose. I was no closer to a CPAP machine than I was before. I had a good cry, then lay in bed in pain for the next 3 days. The details of this event would only become funny in retrospect.

So, now what? My insurance company refused to pay for a second test, even though the first one had been useless. I filed an appeal, describing my experience in finite detail after which a second test was approved and ordered. (This was the first and only time an appeal of mine to an insurance company ever had a positive result. Perhaps my threat to write an article about my experience for the local newspaper had its intended effect!)

This test couldn't have been more different. It was professionally done in the comfort of my own home. In the afternoon, a technician arrived with the equipment. I filled out more papers. He showed me how to connect everything to my body at bedtime, including the telephone hookup to their office where the data would be recorded and evaluated. I was welcome to take any medication necessary to help me sleep. Relief that no strange man was on the other side of my bedroom door and no noise from external "commerce" made sleep quite easy despite all the wires connected to my body.

Unfortunately, after all I'd gone through, the results of the test weren't sufficient to qualify me for a CPAP machine. At that time the requirement was to stop breathing 25 times each hour. I only stopped 17. That meant my insurance company wouldn't cover the cost. Unable to afford the $2,500 price tag, I chose to await another opportunity.

Some months ago, my husband reported an increase in my snoring. After informing my new Kaiser doctor, that opportunity arose. Another professionally-done, at-home sleep study was done. It showed my condition had worsened, and I easily qualified for coverage. Only then did I discover the size of the mask that was part of the equipment I was given to use. As a true claustrophobiac, anything over my face makes me nervous. I seriously doubted my ability to relax enough to sleep while wearing it. Fortunately, they were able to accommodate me with a different version that had only two small tubes for the nostrils, just like getting oxygen. I was delighted that I had slept just fine while wearing it. The problem was that when I awoke I had severe pain and swelling in my face. After looking up my nose, my doctor reported that my breathing passages were unusually narrow. The increased rush of air from the CPAP machine had nowhere to go besides my sinuses. He forecasted more of the same discomfort each night. Sadly, there would be no CPAP machine for me!

Apnea isn't the only sleep problem fibromites have. Many of us suffer from insomnia and frequent awakening as well. Unfortunately, medications that help with falling asleep leave me feeling groggy all the next day. It contributes significantly to my difficulty in getting out of bed. My choices are to sleep all night and most of the next day with the help of medication or not to sleep at all either time. What a choice!

There is an abundance of advice available on the topic of insomnia. Just thinking about it all could keep you awake. Some suggestions work for one person and not for another. Some suggestions will work for you today but not tomorrow.

Here are a few additional things worth trying after you've done all the basic things (known as "sleep hygiene) like refraining from caffeine, increasing your physical activity early in the day, darkening your bedroom, soundproofing as much as possible and limiting alcohol use. These practices may assist with keeping you asleep as well as with falling asleep initially.

Before bed:

- Don't eat after 7 p.m.
- Practice yoga postures in the early evening.
- Use your bedroom exclusively for sleep and sex.
- Always keep a window open at least a little.

- Try a different pillow. (Personally, down works best for me)
- Read a dull book for 20 minutes.
- Consider taking melatonin. (Be aware that it causes depression in some people)
- Drink a glass of warm milk with some cheese or a slice of turkey and some crackers. The protein/carbohydrates combination is said to be relaxing.
- Take a hot bath, shower or sauna before bed. Most experts on the topic agree that a decrease in body temperature at bedtime facilitates sleep.
- Take L-tryptophan or kava.
- Try medical marijuana (if it's legal in your state and you have the required license or recommendation to use it)

After getting in bed:

- Stare at the blackness inside your eyelids. Keep bringing your mind back there when you picture anything else.
- With your eyes closed, look up as you inhale, look down as you exhale. Continue until you fall asleep.
- Take a walk in your mind. Think of a place you haven't been to in a long time. Then picture as many details as you can remember as you stroll along.
- Listen to an iPod turned into a podcast rather than to music.
- Try breathing techniques like Dr. Weil's "relaxing breath" (See More Than Tender Points chapter: Take a Deep Breath)
- Try to watch your breathing rather than control it. (It's more difficult than it sounds, but just

concentrating on trying to do it is in itself relaxing. It erases all the other thoughts that are racing around in your brain and keeping you awake)
- If you aren't asleep after 15 minutes, get up.

If more drastic steps are required, consider the following:

- Dr. H. Ross in his book, <u>Sleep Disorders,</u> recommends pulling circuit breakers to cut all electrical power to the house before bed. Electro-magnetic fields are likely to affect the production of serotonin and melatonin that assist with sleep.
- Keep all electrical devices such as alarm clocks, lamps, CPAP machines, phones, etc. as far from your bed as possible. Three feet is recommended.
- Lose weight if necessary. Obesity contributes to sleep apnea – known to prevent a restful night's sleep.

If none of these techniques work for you either, here are five techniques from Chinese medicine outlined in his book, Secrets to Self Healing by Dr. Maoshing Ni. They are:

1. Acupressure: specifically using your fingertips to press key points on your body to stimulate healing. Two places that are helpful for sleep are
   a. The Inner Gate - which is 3 finger widths above your wrist crease. Apply moderate pressure with your right thumb, holding for 5 minutes and breathing deeply. Repeat on other arm.

b. Bubbling Spring. This spot is on the center of the bottom of the indentation of the ball of your foot. Press with your thumb for 30 seconds, relax for 5, then again for 5 minutes.

2. Jujube seed: According to Dr. Mao, research has shown that this seed strengthens the heart and supports a good night's sleep. It is rich in saponins known to promote relaxation while reducing irritability and anxiety. Typical dose is 500mg/day.

3. Empty your mind before sleep: Try writing in a journal nightly to get worries out of your mind or go even deeper by practicing meditation (See Chapter: Control Your Thoughts)

4. Specific exercise moves: Recommended by GE Hong, the famous Taoist physician from the Han dynasty, these four exercises are for prevention and treatment of insomnia.

    •   Lie on your back, knees bent. Pull your knees toward your chest with your hands and breathe naturally. Hold one minute. Relax. Straighten your legs. Rest your arms at your sides.
    •   Remain on your back. As you inhale, stretch arms above your head. Exhale and bring hands down, massaging your body from your chest to your abdomen. Rest hands at sides. Repeat with each breath for one minute.
    •   Without changing position, make fist with both hands. Place under back as high as you

can toward shoulders, either side of spine. Take three breaths. Reposition fists downward and repeat, moving down every third breath until fists are at waist level. Breathe 5 times here. Place fists either side of tailbone. Breathe 5 more times.

- Lie face down with hands under abdomen. Inhale slowly. Fill abdomen and chest. Feel energy permeate body. Slowly exhale, visualizing everything negative leaving your body. Pause after each exhale to relax muscles. Do for one minute.

5. Taoist sleep position (called Deer Sleep Posture): Turn partway over onto your right side. Bend your right arm at the elbow, palm facing up toward your face. Rest left arm with elbow on hip, hand in front of abdomen. Right leg is straight, left knee bent, rest on mattress in front of right thigh.

Of everything you can do to manage your fibromyalgia symptoms, sleep improvement will probably have the most positive effect. Whether it's an exercise regime, an appropriate medication, an herb or a CPAP machine, it's vitally important to do everything you can to improve your quality of sleep. It will also improve the quality of your life.

Discussion Questions:

> *What causes the worst sleep problems for you?*
> *What techniques do you use to improve insomnia or quality of sleep?*

Chapter 12

In the Mood

W hen you live each and every day with the stress of FM, it doesn't take much to push you over the edge. An upsetting life event occurs (be it a fender-bender, a burned casserole, a computer crash, what have you), it's enough to make most people annoyed for a bit. Pretty quickly they forget it and go on with their lives. For us, it's not so easy. Because stress is cumulative, even small stressors can cause overload.

Symptoms of overload are different for everyone. For some, it could be tears, for others anger. It could also be lowered self-esteem, or even substance abuse. When you have a job, overload is almost inevitable. It takes enormous strength of character to maintain the positive attitude so critical to success when you're battling daily physical symptoms.

Some of us are born fighters. We don't give up easily. We read everything available, consult specialists, practice relaxation techniques and meditation, change our diets. If none of those work, we change doctors, exercise religiously, try the newest medications, and learn self-hypnosis. Nothing is too difficult or too great an effort if it would result in being able to live a more normal life. On and on we go, trying harder and harder. Then one day, the will to fight just can't be mustered any more.

Anyway, that's what happened to me. The stress of my job, in addition to worsening pain and fatigue, cognitive difficulties and IBS made it just too hard to continue. Frightened as I was, I knew I had to make some major changes in my life.

The first major change was to leave my job. It wasn't a decision I arrived at easily. As a widow who'd been left no life insurance, I was my sole source of income. In addition, I had attended college at night while working full time and being a soccer mom to earn the degree that led to the career that I had. My identity was attached to my job, so I struggled against disability for many years. Eventually, my symptoms made the choice for me.

The second major change was to sell my home and move across the country - from the snowy northeast to southern California. As drastic as this was, it was a much less difficult choice to make than leaving my job was. Although I had to sell nearly everything I owned in order to afford the move, I had no regrets. I was moving toward something positive - a home without stairs or the responsibilities of ownership, a climate with no ice to slip on and no snow to shovel, and sunshine: wonderful, glorious sunshine! In retrospect, it was a healthy, cleansing experience. It allowed me to let go of the past and make room for the future in my life.

Although the stress of the move resulted in more pain and fatigue than I'd ever experienced, I was happy. Each day I walked a little, the next day I swam a little. I increased my activity very gradually, but within six months I could hardly remember the wobbly legs that required the use of a cane upon my arrival. On one of my walks, I met a man who would later become my second husband. We bought a little house with a big ocean view, and ever since then I feel like I'm on vacation every day.

And then depression set in. I've learned to recognize it as soon as it appears, but I've yet to learn to prevent it. It's devious. It seeps into your life, usually without warning, and usually when you've settled into a comfortable routine, doing the things you must and maybe even some things you enjoy.

When I'm depressed, getting out of bed in the morning is often an enormous challenge. Here's what I do to prepare for the morning. Just before bedtime I drink 1 or 2 large glasses of water, at least. This way, when I awaken in the morning, I'll have an urgent reason to get up. If you're like me, being roused by your own bladder is much less unpleasant than being roused by an irritating alarm clock.

Another technique I've used is to set the bedroom TV to come on to a news program about 10 minutes before I need to get up. If the volume is sufficiently loud to ignore, I often get interested in the topic being discussed and can be motivated to open at least one eye to see who's talking.

Consider opening your bedroom blinds so that the sun can come in the window in the morning. There's something so natural and non-disturbing about being awakened in this way. After all, the sun is nature's alarm clock. Something to keep in mind, however, is that the skin of our eyelids gets thinner as we age. I find now that I need to wear an eyeshade or I wake up as soon as the sun rises.

If I absolutely need to get up at a specific time, I set my alarm clock and place it across the room. This way I have no choice but to get up to turn it off. This is not to say that I've never hit the snooze bar and stumbled back to bed, but the odds are better that once I'm on my feet and feel nature's call, I'm more inclined to stay up.

Then there's breakfast. This can also be a motivator, especially if you discipline yourself not to eat after dinnertime the night before. Try to relegate some favorite food (like honeydew melon and/or a whole wheat cinnamon bun) as a breakfast-only treat. I've even taped photos of my favorite breakfast foods on my bathroom mirror to remind myself that there's a pleasant experience awaiting me in the kitchen if I stay up and begin the day rather than going back to bed.

Depression presents itself in many forms, only one of which is over-sleeping. The inability to sleep at all is just as common. Feeling irritable, weight changes, cognition problems and physical problems that don't respond to treatment are other indicators.

As soon as the first signs appear (for me it may be lack of interest or insomnia) I quickly assess the amount of exercise I've been doing. The energy it takes just to attend to the necessities of life often robs me of the energy required to exercise regularly. Without exercise, depression is an all too frequent visitor. Seclusion is the other culprit. For me, writing can be compulsive and isolating, but it's part of who I am. Socializing takes more effort, but it is vitally important for my sense of well being. This may not be true for you. Everyone is different.

Positive affirmations are helpful, too. Before I go to bed, I repeat several times, "I wake up feeling refreshed and eager to start the day." First thing in the morning I write my goals for the day, again in the form of positive affirmations, such as "I feel healthy and strong," or "I exercise for half an hour every day," or "I arrive at my appointments on time."

Even more powerful is making the generic statement, "Something wonderful will happen to me today." This is something I have taped to my mirror. As I lie in bed awaiting sleep, I try to think of anything wonderful that did happen that day. I'm often surprised and grateful for how many items I can list.

Dietary changes such as restricting sugar, alcohol and caffeine can also be helpful to your mood. Nutritional deficiencies can contribute to depression. Because the soil our food is grown in today is often depleted of necessary minerals, even a healthy diet doesn't always include everything our bodies need. Omega-3 is one nutrient often in short supply. It is found predominantly in flax seeds and fish oils. A cure for your depression may be as close as the nearest health food store. A supplement may be all you need.

Some people read spiritually uplifting books when they're depressed. I would like to, but I can't. My brain just doesn't process the words. This happens to be another fairly common symptom of depression. I could read the same sentence a dozen times and still not know what I read. Thankfully, we now have audiobooks. With a little motivation, I can usually push myself to listen to something – even if it's not spiritual.

Another idea is to use music as therapy. Start by playing some really slow, dark music to match your present mood, something like the second movement of Beethoven's third symphony. After a few minutes, progress to something a bit more upbeat, maybe a Mozart violin concerto or a Sinatra ballad. Then move on to something a little peppier, like your favorite jazz artist, and so on. The idea is that your mood will become happier as the music becomes happier. I've done this many times, and it has worked for me on several occasions. (Hint: Changing stations on the radio or music stations on your cable TV can achieve the same result.)

I've jokingly renamed FM the "Cancellation Disease". You make plans to go somewhere with someone when you're feeling o.k. Then, when the time comes, you're suddenly experiencing some symptom that prevents you from leaving the house. Being sociable is out of the question. So you call and cancel. Or you're invited to a party, accept the invitation and then cancel an hour before it begins. There are just so many times you can cancel before the invitations stop coming.

It's important to have someone to confide in, but you don't want that person to be your spouse or significant other. That person has enough to endure just by living with you. Hearing about every unpleasant symptom you're experiencing is too big a burden for one person to bear. Support groups are a great solution, but unfortunately they normally meet only once a month.

If at all possible, find yourself an FM buddy in your support group or chat room and make contact with each other a couple of times a week. Have yourselves a real pity party. Cry if you want to. But limit the time to 15 or 20 minutes each. It can be physically exhausting to share someone else's pain. It can also add to your own depression if it goes on too long. Try to end the conversation with a couple of upbeat suggestions for each other.

It's very common for people with FM to experience anxiety in addition to depression. They both involve negative thinking. Anxiety is the fear that something bad is going to happen. Depression is the belief that life is already bad and often fosters feelings of hopelessness.

The good news is that they are both treatable. Therapists or social workers who practice CBT (cognitive behavioral therapy) can be extremely useful in helping you to understand how your thoughts are affecting your feelings, making you either anxious or depressed. They can suggest techniques for changing those thoughts. Quite often, when you cure your anxiety, you cure your depression as well. A psychiatrist I met feels they are the exact same disorder – only at different ends of the spectrum she refers to as "mood disorder".

The most important thing to know about depression is not to ignore it. If your self-help attempts don't work, see your doctor without delay. There are many classes of drugs on the market that are very effective - especially when combined with increased exercise, CBT and nutritional supplementation.

Your challenge is to find what works best for you. It will take some time and effort because each person's body is very different, but a good doctor will be willing to work with you no matter how long it takes. If you get no help from the first doctor you see, search out another one. The right one for you is available, and it's worth the effort to find that person. Your happiness is dependent upon it.

I make it a practice to see my therapist any time the remedies I usually employ aren't working, and/or my depression or anxiety persists for more than a week or two. After a couple of sessions, the cause usually becomes apparent, and then I can start working on the cure. However, there have been times when CBT didn't work for me, and I needed an anti-depressant medication as well. With all my side effects, that's always my very last resort.

An important word of warning:

If you ever experience suicidal thoughts, contact a doctor, psychologist or therapist immediately. If yours isn't available, go to the nearest Emergency Room.

Here's what the late Dr. Norman Vincent Peale had to say about depression in his classic book called Imaging: Imagine you are suffering from depression.

Picture that horrible word spelled out in gigantic letters on a sign on a mountaintop. Each letter is ten feet tall and can be seen at night for miles. Now imagine the first two and the eighth letter were suddenly extinguished. What's left?" PRESS ON.

Discussion Questions:

Are there specific triggers that cause episodes of either depression or anxiety for you?
Have you tried CBT and how successful was it?
Do your moods correspond to your pain level?

Chapter 13

Always Too Tired

Tired is a relative term. It means different things to different people. To a runner, it may be the inability to finish a marathon. To a working mother of small children it may be the inability to bathe squirming little bodies after a tough day on the job. But no other "tired" bares any resemblance to the profound fatigue experienced by nearly every FM sufferer I've ever met, with the possible exception of someone suffering from a severe case of influenza or the after effects of chemotherapy. There are many theories why we fibromites suffer this debilitating symptom – two of which are non-restorative sleep (due to conditions such as untreated sleep apnea which results in a reduction of REM sleep) and the co-existence of chronic fatigue syndrome.

Whatever the reason, just walking from the bedroom to the kitchen is a challenge for me on some days. Climbing a flight of stairs is out of the question. Even holding my head up can be daunting. So, what to do?

You rest. Yes. That's all you can do. You cancel or reschedule every activity you had planned and concentrate on getting through the day. If you think long and hard you will realize that your overactivity of the day before is likely responsible for the way you feel today. You may not have done a lot (as measured by the rest of the population) but for you it was clearly too much. It takes years to learn this lesson. But one day the fact that prevention is the only cure for this condition finally becomes embedded in your brain.

Whenever we feel well enough, there's a mile-long list of things that need doing, and an even longer list of things that would be fun to do. And who doesn't want to have fun? More importantly, there is exercise to be done. So, you have all these things to do and only a limited amount of energy. The solution is to live by a schedule, one you've tailored to your own capabilities.

You begin by making two lists every day first thing in the morning. The first list includes all the things you need to get done for the day (and perhaps a few things you would like to do). The second list contains the same items but considers the two essentials that can make the difference between leading a productive life and not.

The first essential is pacing. The second is exercise. Pacing is basically resting before you feel tired. It sounds easy enough, but it's especially difficult for those of us who are tired much of the time and want to make the most of our occasional good days. It's most challenging for the over-achievers among us. Exercise is the other essential, even if it's only stretching. Without these two items, your chances of ever successfully completing your to-do list are very slim indeed.

The thing about including exercise on your list is that after this becomes an integral part of your day, you will notice an improvement in your energy level. The more you do, the more you can do. If walking is your exercise of choice, over time you'll be able to extend your 5 minute walk to 6 minutes, then 8 and so on. Your goal should be 30 minutes, but don't be in a hurry to get there. It's very important not to make the increases too quickly. If you do, you'll find yourself too tired to go on with your day and accomplish nothing at all. Even worse, the next day you're apt to feel no better. In any case, you're likely to become discouraged and go back to doing nothing at all.

My advice is to maintain your current level of exercise for at least 2 weeks or until you feel really comfortable with it before moving up another minute or two. Then remain at that level for a week or two before any further increases. Remember that getting started is the difficult part until it becomes a habit. It's been said that it takes 21 days to form a habit, so be patient. Once you incorporate exercise into your life, you'll feel incomplete without it.

Just don't expect to see miracles. Fibromyalgia has changed your body; your expectations must change as well. Remember the tortoise and the hare. Slow and steady wins the race.

Now back to pacing. A list with pacing considered will alternate tasks between those that require physical exertion and those that can be done while seated or lying down. You'll be pleasantly surprised at how many of the things you do on a routine basis can be done in a seated or prone position. I make phone calls lying on my back, peel potatoes and stir things on the stove while seated on a stool, and fold clothes while sitting on my bed with my feet up.

My list always includes a 15 minute stretch in the morning and a similar one in the afternoon. It also includes a half hour rest period after each one during which time I lie on my back with a pillow under my knees and a nightshade over my eyes. Then I either catnap or meditate or do a little of each.

Believe it or not, you can adhere to such a schedule and still maintain a clean and tidy house, eat 3 meals a day, spend time with a friend or do something else you enjoy. For me, that's writing. You may not have as much energy as you once had, but you can still live a productive life. You just need a little practice in adhering to a schedule that will allow you to do so.

Being organized is a big plus when it comes to fatigue. If you have a task to do, such as opening the day's mail, assemble all the necessary tools before you begin. This saves much up and down and walking to and fro to retrieve needed objects. A lesson I learned from a Time Management class I attended while still working in corporate America is to handle each piece of paper only once. It's a real challenge at first. But, of all the ways I know to save energy, I consider this to be the most effective.

Here's how I put it into practice: After the mailman comes, I move my wastebasket next to my filing cabinet next to my desk, pull up a chair, have phone, paper and pen nearby. With letter opener in hand, I begin my attack. Advertising goes directly into the garbage. Anything worth saving is filed in my file cabinet. Bills either get paid immediately (if I have the funds available), or they can go into files numbered with the days of the month. If a bill needs to be paid or some action needs to be taken on the 15th of the month, I drop it in file #15 of the files I have labeled 1 thru 31. If it's a receipt for something I purchased, it goes in the file marked purchases for the year, most recent in front (just in case it needs to be returned). If it's something I don't understand, my phone is at the ready to call and get the issue resolved. Not only does this process save physical energy, it also fosters peace of mind. Seeing a mountain of paper that needs attention can, in itself, be fatiguing. Having dealt with it all when it arrived can create be enormous relief.

Another helpful technique is to divide large tasks into smaller portions so that you can cross something off your to-do list as being "done". It will give you a needed sense of accomplishment even if you don't do everything you wanted to do that day. And forgive yourself if you don't have enough energy to complete your list. What you don't finish today, you can always do tomorrow. With planning and perseverance you can do whatever you'd like to do. You'll just learn to do it on your own terms.

Just as I did, you'll learn little tricks along the way for preserving the energy you have. One little thing I've done that sounds really insignificant is to adhere to a policy of only buying clothes that have pockets. This way, I carry a purse only on those occasions when it's absolutely necessary. Tiny changes like this will make a significant difference in the amount of energy you have available. Do whatever you can to make your life easier. The result will be an increased ability to do the things you really want to do.

By using pacing and scheduling exercise you can still have goals and a reasonable expectation of accomplishing them. And that's a very uplifting feeling. It takes a great deal of discipline, especially at first, and particularly when you're feeling poorly. But I promise you it's worth the effort.

As in all things related to fibromyalgia, you must listen to your body. If, on a particularly bad day, you feel completely unable to do anything at all, you must learn not to push on, but to just go lay down. It's possible you'll feel revived later in the day. At that time you may feel capable of doing a few things - or maybe you won't. In any case, you'll be living life on your own terms. Remember that compassion for yourself is as important as pacing or exercise or anything else that you do.

Discussion Questions:

> *Do you follow a schedule?*
> *Have you incorporated pacing into your life?*
> *What about exercise?*
> *Have any of these made a difference in your level of fatigue?*
> *Does anything else not mentioned here improve your fatigue level?*

Chapter 14

Possible Side Effects

Those three words "Possible Side Effects" always make me chuckle. If they only knew!! For me and for many fibromites, there's no "possible" about it. Our sensitive bodies react to everything, from drugs to foods to body lotion! With us, the question isn't, "Will there be side effects?" The question is "Will the side effects be worse than the problem being treated?"

Years ago, very few over-the-counter medications were kept in the typical home. When I was growing up, our options were limited to aspirin, Bufferin or Anacin for pain, Alka-Seltzer or Pepto-Bismol for stomach problems and Kaopectate for diarrhea. Of those, I could only tolerate the Kaopectate. The other 3 made my stomach hurt, my esophagus burn or made me nauseous. I learned early on not to complain about pain.

If I were sick enough to need a doctor, one came to the house and gave me a shot of penicillin. I'm suspicious of the effect all that penicillin had on my body. As a child, I was sick a lot!

Over the years physicians often refused to believe that the unpleasant symptoms I was having were side effects of the drugs they prescribed. They believed I had the symptoms all right, (It's difficult to ignore a patient who is vomiting in your office.) but they flatly refused to believe the symptoms were the result of the medication they had prescribed. It was always attributed to having the flu.

If I were a braver person or a masochist, I'd volunteer to participate in drug trials as the token fibromyalgiac. I'm concerned about how differently we react and about how dangerous that difference may ultimately be. In recent separate studies done for men and women on the sleep aid, Ambien, the optimum dose for women was only half of that for men. I believe a third category is needed for people with FM. I actually did participate in one drug trial for just that reason. It was for an IBS drug. The trial was terminated after several participants died. I decided I would let someone else be the guinea pig next time

Speaking of side effects: My experience with hormone replacement therapy (HRT) was particularly unpleasant. Each and every one gave me horrific headaches, stomach cramps and nausea. Even reducing the dosage by three-fourths didn't help. Estrace cream was the best and the worst. After 3 months of using one-quarter of the recommended dose, my symptoms finally went away. That's the good news.

The bad news is that the estrogen in Estrace aggravated the stones that had lain dormant in my gall bladder for many years (according to my surgeon). Pain after every meal radiated from below my right ribcage to my shoulder and back. In addition, I had constant, painful indigestion, and heart palpitations so severe that the noise of it prevented me from sleeping at night. When the results of a sonogram showed lots of small stones in my gall bladder, I had surgery to remove it right away. I didn't like the possibility that one of them might lodge in the bile duct necessitating emergency surgery wherever I might be.

Note: In case you ever need to have it done, gall bladder removal (aka laparoscopic cholecystectomy) is a very simple procedure in most cases these days. Only three inch-long incisions are necessary. The procedure takes about 20 minutes. You go home 3 hours after you arrive at the hospital. Aside from discomfort on the right side for the next several days, it's really quite painless.

The only problem I had was with (surprise, surprise) side effects from drugs. In hindsight, I remember feeling a little hyper and having trouble sleeping after previous injections of Torradol. But because I'd had Torradol so many times before, I just chalked those symptoms up to situational conditions.

I should have known better. The post-surgical Torradol injection I received in the hospital for pain caused itching, reflux and heart palpitations. My surgeon refused to believe the Torradol caused those symptoms and sent me home with more. When will I learn? When the pain became severe, I took one more, and two hours later the itching became overwhelming, my eyelids swelled nearly shut, and I was awake for another entire night. Forty-eight hours post surgery I'd only slept two hours.

Desperate, I called the surgeon again, who finally understood there was a problem with his drug of choice. This time he prescribed Darvocet. It worked wonderfully, calming the itching, the pain, the swollen eyelids, the reflux, and the palpitations. I slept for the next two days.

I've concluded that nearly half the suffering in my life has been self-induced. It was caused by something I ingested - like a drug or a vitamin or a supplement or even food. Over the years, I'm sure I missed more days from school and from work due to side effects from medication than I ever did from illness. The thing I regret most is that I waited so long to begin my practice of keeping a record of what I took and what it did to me. Don't make the same mistake I did. Keep an accurate and up-to-date paper trail and keep it with you at all times! (See Chapter 21) WRITE IT DOWN

Here's another tip: If a doctor wants you to try a new medication, ASK FOR SAMPLES! Most doctors see drug salesmen and receive free samples. The reason they have them is to give to their patients. The drug company's goal is to establish a pattern that you will continue after the samples run out and you begin having prescriptions filled. The beauty of samples for patients like us with a high risk of intolerance is that they can save you a whole lot of time, money, and effort (like standing in line at the drugstore while feeling weak and unwell). As with many other aspects of life, you don't get if you don't ask. So, always ask for samples.

If your doctor has no samples, ask your pharmacist to fill only a portion of the prescription until you know if you can tolerate it. Just because a prescription is written for 30 pills doesn't mean you have to purchase the 30 all at once - unless your insurance will only pay that way.

If it's a drug your insurance doesn't cover, be sure your doctor knows that. There are often equivalent drugs he can prescribe instead – or he may then be motivated to find some samples for you. If you have no insurance coverage for drugs, purchase only enough for 3 days to start. You can always go back and get the remainder.

Because my body is so sensitive, half or less of the normally prescribed dose is all it takes to be effective for me (if I can tolerate it at all). A pediatric dose is often all I can handle. When it comes to narcotic pain relievers, however, several studies including one by Daniel Clauw, M.D. et. al. published in the Sept. 2007 edition of The Journal of Neuroscience concluded that due to decreased opioid receptor availability, fibromyalgiacs need more not less narcotic medications than other people do to be effective. If you ever need surgery, be sure that both your surgeon and your anesthesiologist know that you have FM.

Here's a bit of essential advice: Never assume that because you took a drug successfully once that you can take it again. This isn't necessarily true. Side effects or allergies can develop at any time. Always be alert to the signs that you may be having a negative reaction.

I took a sulfa drug at least once before I developed an allergy to it that landed me in the hospital. On this occasion, after a rash appeared on my neck, my throat began to close, and my entire body gradually went numb. Fortunately, the phone was right next to me when it began. By the time the paramedics arrived, the rash had spread to my chest, my limbs wouldn't move, and I was too short of breath to get up to answer the door. Because of this experience, I learned to notify someone before I begin taking a new drug. When I lived alone, I made certain there was easy access to my house. Fire departments may or may not force their way in as the dedicated men who arrived at my home did. A broken door is much preferable to death.

Don't expect all of a drug's potential side effects to be listed on the bottle or even printed on the write-up inside the box. These effects were observed in normal people, not in people with FM. Let your body be your guide. If you notice anything unusual at all, call your doctor or your pharmacist.

Another thing to consider is that the generic version of a drug you've been successfully taking may be quite different from the brand name drug. There are also differences between generic versions by different manufacturers of the same drug. One company in particular produces a generic version of morphine sulfate that has absolutely no effect on the nerve pain I occasionally experience, whereas another generic brand works just fine. There have even been a couple of occasions when I had to pay the difference between the cost of the generic drug (which my insurance covered) and the cost of the brand name drug (which was not covered) because only the brand name drug solved the problem for me without causing side effects.

I've encountered several FM patients over the years who cannot tolerate any pharmaceuticals at all. Out of necessity they have turned to Eastern (Chinese) medicine. They choose Naturopathic physicians or herbalists instead of conventional doctors or a combination of both. The older I get and the more side effects I endure, the more inviting Eastern medicine is to me. See more about this in the Chapter on Herbal Remedies.

One last word on this topic: It's important to trust your physician but it's equally important to trust yourself and your knowledge of your own body - especially when it comes to Side Effects.

Discussion Questions:

> *Is your body sensitive to medications?*
> *What type of reactions have you experienced?*
> *How soon did they subside?*
> *Was there a substitute for the drug available?*

Chapter 15

Aquatic Therapy May be Hazardous to Your Health

Physicians frequently recommend warm water exercise for the treatment of FM. But before you dive in, I'd like to share my experience with you. It was definitely not what I was expecting. There are perils in the pool, and you should be aware of what they are.

First, let me say that if done in moderation, warm water exercise is among the most effective treatments for FM pain and is utilized around the world. Study results published in Barcelona's Medicina Clinica (Dec 2013) reported improvements in sleep quality, anxiety, pain and other fibromyalgia symptoms from a therapy known as Aquatic Biodanza (translation: freestyle dancing done in warm water).

The buoyancy and warmth of the water makes movement of any kind easier, producing less trauma to painful joints and making it possible to exercise longer without fatigue. Having said that, keep in mind that not every experience will produce the same results. You must pay attention to the details!

For many years, at the encouragement of my rheumatologist, I swam laps 2-3 times a week at my local YMCA on my way home from work. The pool was maintained at 85 degrees Fahrenheit, cool enough to encourage energetic movement but warm enough not to increase my pain. Any cooler caused my muscles to contract and my joints to ache for several hours and sometimes into the next day as well. I learned to carefully monitor the temperature and forego my swim when the water felt too cold for me. Swimming kept my fibro symptoms in check for years. It tired me sufficiently so that I slept and functioned with a minimum of medication - usually just a small dose of a muscle relaxant at bedtime.

Over the course of many years, my FM symptoms worsened. I could no longer work, and swimming laps became much too strenuous for me. I tried water aerobics, but that was even worse. Then I heard about the Arthritis Foundation's Aquatics Program specifically for FM. It was held at a pool heated to 90 degrees. This sounded like the perfect solution: exercise tailored to my needs and no more cold water to worry about!

The class was paced for varying levels of ability. Delighted to be back in the water, the first time I attended the class I participated fully only at a minimum level, but for the entire 60-minutes. All was well until it was time to get out of the pool. Suddenly I realized that my legs wouldn't work. I couldn't climb up the steps to get out of the water.

Thinking I was just more tired than I realized, I leaned against the side of the pool and waited a few minutes before I tried again. The second attempt was even worse. My legs collapsed like two wet noodles. I was totally embarrassed (not to mention frightened) as I watched the pool area empty. How could I get out of the pool? How could I drive home?

Fortunately, the Arthritis Foundation sponsored this class, and the pool was equipped with a lift for patients who needed assistance getting in and out of the water. One of the instructors finally noticed me clinging to the side of the pool. I explained my problem, and they quickly hoisted me out. Relieved, I felt confident that after sitting for a while I'd regain my strength, get dressed and go home. However, this was not to be. Soon it became apparent that my arms weren't working either. Eventually an ambulance was called, and three members of my fibro support group (May they be blessed forever.) accompanied me in my wet bathing suit to the local Emergency Room. By this time, my body was shaking from head to toe. It wasn't from the cold. I was scared to death!

Every negative scenario I could imagine flooded my mind. I pictured being forever in a wheelchair in my multi-level house, completely dependent upon other people to fulfill my every need. I was too frightened to cry.

The hospital admitted me for testing. I had all the classic symptoms of multiple sclerosis. Thankfully, every neurological test they performed showed negative results. For five days, I languished in that hospital bed, unable to raise a hand or a foot, only able to turn my head, the only part of my body which hadn't been submerged in the water. The prospect of going home where I lived alone was as daunting as being unable to move.

On the 6th day, they delivered the "good news/good news" to me. The "good" news was that they found nothing wrong with me. The further "good" news (but it sure didn't feel good to me) was that I was being discharged the next day.

The prospect of returning to my three-level house when I could only walk a few feet using a walker was just as frightening as my lack of strength. I lived alone and had no family in town. My really close friends were people I'd worked with for nearly 20 years. Since I'd left on disability 9 months earlier, I was seeing them less and less. I couldn't imagine how I'd care for my own needs alone.

Have you ever heard it said that you don't know who your friends are until you really need them? Believe it! My fibromyalgia support group was truly supportive (delivering meals and boosting my morale). My neighbors (some of whom I hadn't seen since my then 30 yr. old son had been a cub scout) showed up at my door with food. They also did my laundry, my banking, my cooking and my grocery shopping.

For the first two weeks I slept in the downstairs of my multi-level home on the family room couch. During this time a physical therapist and an occupational therapist helped me function and regain strength. I could maneuver pretty well on the first floor using a walker on wheels that my insurance company provided. Eventually I was able to navigate my stairs again, down once in the morning and up once at night. It was a major production each time, but it was do-able.

This was the most frightening experience of my life. I share it with you now to save you from the same fate. Yes, warm water exercise is wonderful therapy for fibromyalgia. But, it must be tailored for every individual. The water temperature may be too warm for some or the class may last too long. Each person's tolerance is very different. For me, 60 minutes in 90 degree water was way more than I could tolerate and resulted in a complete muscle collapse. However, there were many other fibromites in that class who had been attending that class every week for years. They did just fine from day one.

My advice is to ease into any exercise program gradually, especially warm water programs. Because they are deceptively easy to do, the tendency is to do more than you can tolerate. Never, ever stay in a very warm pool or tub for more than 10 minutes until you know how your body will react. I usually live by the mantra: "Listen to your body", but this case is an exception. Being in warm water can feel luxurious and painless for a very long time – sometimes much longer than your muscles can endure.

Use even more caution with hot tubs or spas, which are normally kept at over 100 degrees. They may feel like heaven on earth, and they can do wonderful things for sore, achy muscles. But don't let a relaxing soak precipitate a day in bed. This is truly a case where less is more.

If you don't wish to participate in a formal aquatics class, you can always do water exercises on your own. However, I would caution you to keep a watchful eye on the water temperature and on the clock. If the temperature feels comfortable to you, begin with 5-10 minutes at a time and remain at that level for several days until you're certain the desired effect is being achieved. Then, and only then, move up a couple of minutes. At this point, it will be more effort to wriggle in and out of your bathing suit than the exercise you do in the water. Even so, resist the temptation to do more until you're certain that what you're doing is beneficial for you.

I have included pool exercises in Appendix D which also may be found on my website at www.fmspubs.com. These exercises were recommended by the Arthritis Foundation, and I have found them extremely effective when done in moderation. You can make a copy of the pages, put them in a plastic zip-lock bag and take them with you to the pool.

Just walking in chest-deep water is terrific exercise. It is also a good warm-up and should be done for about 5 minutes before progressing to more vigorous activity such as an aquatics class or lap swimming. You can use different muscles by first walking forward, then walking backward, then walking from side to side.

You can do most any stretch in the water that you can do on dry land. Just remember to do it slowly and to avoid repetitive motion. It's important to keep your arms in the water, too. Lifting them puts a lot of stress on your shoulder and neck muscles, places that are particularly subject to FM pain. As with any exercise you do, concentrate mainly on stretching, never on the number of repetitions. This will increase your range of motion and make your daily activities easier to perform.

Lastly, here's a tip I learned from a medical advice column in the local newspaper that has nothing to do with fibromyalgia, but has everything to do with enjoying the water. For those of us who are prone to "swimmer's ear", mix equal parts white vinegar and rubbing alcohol in a small empty pill bottle. Warm slightly by holding the closed bottle under hot tap water. Put 2 drops in each ear after swimming, one ear at a time. Leave for half a minute, then tilt your head and let it drain out. This helps keep the ears dry and prevents itching and infection.

So, go ahead and get your feet (and body) wet. Aquatic therapy can be wonderful. Keep in mind the precautions mentioned above, and remember, as with any other activity for those with FM, moderation is the key.

Discussion Questions:

> *Have you tried warm water therapy for your FM?*
> *Did you go to a class? Where?*
> *What were your results?*

Chapter 16

More About Exercise

Whenever we feel well enough, there's a mile-long list of things that need doing, and an even longer list of things that would be fun to do. And who can resist having fun? So, on we go, doing and doing, getting more and more tired, thereby eliminating the possibility of exercise from the day's activities.

Following my disastrous experience in the overly-warm pool, I turned to yoga, the next most commonly recommended exercise for those with FM. There are at least 19 schools of Yoga, each requiring a different degree of physical effort, making some more suitable for fibromites than others.

Hatha yoga is the foundation of all Yoga styles. It is a combination of postures, breathing techniques and meditation. It has become very popular in this country as a source of exercise and stress management. For that reason, most classes advertised are likely to be in the Hatha style. With its pretzel-like poses it tends to focus on perfecting the physical form and is quite challenging. I would opt for a less strenuous form.

Two schools that are more appropriate for FM sufferers are Kripalu and Kundalini. Kripalu yoga (sometimes referred to as the Yoga of consciousness) focuses on developing physical and spiritual well being.

Kundalini yoga is a combination of meditation and yoga. After practicing this form myself for several years, it would be my first choice for FM sufferers.

Be very wary of Yoga classes offered at health clubs. They are often a combination of yoga and strength training and are much too strenuous for beginners and especially for people with FM. A discussion with the instructor prior to beginning any yoga program is essential. Experienced instructors are accustomed to dealing with health limitations and will modify postures for you accordingly.

Yoga is truly non-competitive and teaches awareness of the body. Regular gentle practice for even a few minutes a day can produce very big changes. The body becomes more toned, and the muscles lose some of the tightness that increases FM pain. Try to incorporate it into your daily routine - like brushing your teeth. It's easier to remember if you do it first thing in the morning or at bedtime each day.

When I moved from NY to California, I left my Kripalu yoga instructor behind and lost the motivation to do my daily practice. I think I was beginning to tire of it as well after having practiced daily for 5 years. That's the bad news.

The good news is that I found what I consider to be an even better exercise for FM. It is called Qi (pronounced "chee") Gong. Although Qi Gong originated from a 3,000 year old Chinese religious practice, it is used in this country to strengthen or balance the body's flow of energy in order to promote healing. It is also an excellent relaxation technique and is less strenuous than Tai Chi.

The particular Qi Gong practice I learned is called Eight Pieces of Brocade. There are eight basic poses that become routine after doing them a number of times. Each one stretches a different part of the body, something that is essential for tight FM muscles. It heals by aligning breath, movement, and meditation.

The best way to learn Qi Gong is to take a class. The instructor can make certain you're doing the poses correctly. If there are no classes available, turn to the internet. There are many examples on YouTube that you can watch and follow. Because it will be new, it will be a challenge to both watch and do at first, but in time it will become familiar. After finding a YouTube video that looks possible to do and to follow, concentrate on learning just one new pose each week. Play the video over and over, until you feel confident that you know it. Take a few notes or draw a crude picture to remind yourself what each pose looks like after you've learned it. Each pose has a name, but I wouldn't waste my time trying to remember them all. It's more important to learn to do the pose correctly.

Physical therapists often recommend tai chi for fibromyalgia. The slow, gentle movements are purported to soothe stiff muscles and reduce pain. Unfortunately, the repetition required in the learning process isn't factored into the total exercise. As a result, my first attempt at tai chi was anything but healing. The day after the first class I was barely able to get out of bed. Everything hurt, and I was completely exhausted. How could something so good for me be so painful?

The answer was apparent to me once I understood that even the gentlest motion done repetitively can cause pure agony in people with FM. Were I to try tai chi again, I would speak with the instructor before the class and explain my repetitive motion issue. Then I could do much less than the rest of the class without feeling embarrassed and would probably have better albeit slower results.

Having to single myself out in that manner has been a very difficult aspect of having FM for me. It took a long time and lots of mental anguish before I felt comfortable making excuses for myself. Pointing out my limitations was a real downer when I spent so much time and energy trying to be like everyone else.

Another excellent form of exercise for fibromyalgia is walking. Anyone can walk. Right? Just be careful if you haven't done it for a while. When my health-conscious employer encouraged physical activity each day at lunchtime, I felt confident beginning a walking program with my also sedentary co-workers. Our plan was to walk just under a mile at a moderate pace, stopping to rest about half way through. It sounded simple enough, but I only lasted for 3 days. On the 4th day, I awoke with an excruciatingly painful muscle spasm in my right calf. It kept me home taking painkillers and applying moist heat for the next several days. I reported that I had the flu. How else could I explain that 3 days of the same walking that so many others had done along with me caused me so much misery? For a fibromyalgia walking program, speed and distance are not important. Stretching your muscles is the important part.

Only later did I learn that physical therapists recommend stretching as a prerequisite to doing any exercise, including walking. The benefits include reducing muscle tension, increasing flexibility and preventing injuries such as the muscle strain that I experienced. I've been cautioned to ease slowly into any stretch, to keep breathing, and not to hold my breath. The goal is to increase oxygen as well as blood flow to the muscles you're about to use. Upper body stretches should be held for 15 seconds. Lower body stretches for 30 seconds. Repeat each stretch two times.

If I haven't been walking regularly, I now do a few gentle calf stretches before I begin. Here's how: With toes about 24 inches from the wall, take a large step back with one leg. Using the wall for balance and keeping both heels on the floor, bend the front leg while keeping the back leg straight. Hold this position for a few seconds, but do not bounce. Do the same with the other leg. Repeat several times.

Remember to begin walking slowly and to stop before you feel tired. If you are suffering from severe fatigue, you can still walk. Begin by doing very little at one time. A park where there are benches is a good place to start. Use each bench as a goal. Walk from one bench to the next, then sit down and rest. Walk to the next bench, then sit to rest again. I did this when I first moved to California. In addition to meeting many interesting people (including my second husband) while sitting on those benches, I could also measure my progress when I was able to skip a bench or two as the weeks went by. The key is not to push yourself past your capability. Only do a little until you're very comfortable with it. Then do a little more. And rest after whatever you do.

Although walking doesn't require any expensive equipment, a good pair of shoes is a MUST. Muscles and joints can be injured if you're not wearing shoes that absorb impact. Running shoes are especially good for walking. They have great support and plenty of cushioning in the heel. But don't try to fit them yourself. Go to a store that specializes in athletic shoes. They have knowledgeable employees who can find the perfect shoe for you. It may be a pricey purchase, but consider it an investment in your health. Personally, I have found the Brooks Mogo, the SAS walking shoe and the TEVA Circuit Walker Sandal to be the best choices for me. They have the most cushioning in the heel which must be where I concentrate my stride. These are particularly good for my foot because I have a very high arch. Your needs will probably be very different. But only an experienced shoe fitter can tell you that.

If you haven't already, you will soon discover that healthy people (This includes exercise instructors.) often have a difficult time taking FM seriously. It's because most FM sufferers look perfectly healthy. And we're usually quite content to let people think that we're fine when we're not. The unfortunate reality of FM is that we're very different. But with a few accommodations in the right places we can do most of what the rest of the world is doing. Exercising just happens to be one area in which we need a little special consideration.

In summary, here are the basic facts about fibromyalgia and exercise:

First, we MUST exercise. Inactivity is our worst enemy. In healthy people, muscles relax and rejuvenate during REM (Rapid Eye Movement) sleep. People with FM get very little REM sleep so our muscles rarely relax. Without stretching and exercise, we'd be much more stiff and sore each morning than we already are.

Second, exercise must be tailored to our needs. Don't be fooled by programs designed by the Arthritis Foundation for people with other forms of arthritis. Those programs are full of repetitive movements that can be really harmful for us. If you choose to participate in a formal exercise program of any kind, do yourself a favor and let the instructor know at the beginning that you will be modifying the course to fit your FM needs.

Third, (and most difficult to do), is to rest before you feel tired. If necessary, exercise 10 minutes less in order to rest 10 minutes more. Remember that the after-effects of overdoing won't likely be felt until the next day.

Last but not least: Many symptoms of FM can actually be caused by lack of exercise. Weak muscles may be the result of disuse, lack of stimulation and deconditioning. The solution can be strengthening exercises, done slowly and sparingly at first but done regularly. Fatigue, low energy and depression may also be the result of deconditioning and inactivity.

Our overall sense of well being can be greatly increased once we embark on a regular exercise regime. It doesn't need to be aerobic, although that would be a wonderful goal to work toward. The important thing is to get yourself up and moving. The old adage that "if you don't use it, you lose it" is true. The more you sit, the less able you are to get up and go. Inexpensive step counters are available in many places these days. Or download a free app called Stepz on your phone. Keeping a daily count can be an interesting experiment. You'll see how or if your number of daily steps corresponds with your symptoms.

If someone tells you that you must increase your heart rate for your exercise to be beneficial, don't believe it. Rheumatologists have assured me that for someone with fibromyalgia, exercising regularly is far more important than exercising aerobically. Restrict yourself to what your body can handle. Never push yourself past your comfort zone. Your goal should not be to "feel the burn". It should be to "feel no pain".

Discussion Questions:

> *What kinds of exercise do you do?*
> *Do you do daily stretching?*
> *Do you see differences in how you feel if you do or do not stretch or exercise?*

Chapter 17

Simple Pleasures

A good friend once told me, "I know we'll never have a lot of money, and I'm all right with that. Our wealth is in our children." To this day, she savors every day of their lives as well as her own. She truly enjoys the "simple pleasures" she has. If I were asked the best way to enjoy life despite having fibromyalgia, I'd say, "Learn to enjoy the simple pleasures." The most wonderful thing about them is that most cost very little and others are absolutely free!

Here are just a few:

Sunsets:

When was the last time you watched the sun go down? No matter where you live, there's a place close by that has a nice view of this cost-free, heart-lifting phenomenon. If you live on a hill as I do, you can just go out in your own back yard. Where I lived before, there was a park near my home which had a small lake and a nice view. I watched from there. Make it a daily ritual. If you've had a bad day, you can celebrate its ending. If you've had a good day, you can give thanks and pray for another. At the very least, you have something to look forward to each evening. I've heard sunrises are also quite spectacular, although I can't speak from personal experience. Mornings are so difficult for me that I've seen very few in my lifetime. Those were only because I hadn't been to sleep yet.

Baths:

A warm bath in itself is a pleasure, especially if your muscles are sore. But you can make it even more special by pouring yourself your favorite drink, turning on some soothing music and, of course, lighting a couple of candles. When I was still working, I looked forward to this nightly ritual all day long.

Music:

Experiment with all kinds of music and find the style that really speaks to you. Public libraries have all kinds that you can borrow for any kind of music player you have. If you have none, try listening to a different music station on the radio or TV each day until you find something you really enjoy. Make a real effort to find something that soothes your soul. It's very useful on bad days.

If music inspires you to dance, even better. I enjoy Richard Simmons' "Dancing to the Oldies" myself, and I get up and dance along when I feel well enough. If you feel the urge, be sure to wear your walking shoes when you dance. You need the shock absorption to protect your knees, ankles and hips. If you can't dance, you can sway to the music.

Nature:

Before I moved to California, I thought gardening was a huge chore. Nearly everything I planted in Central New

York either froze to death in the winter snow or withered and died in the August heat. Living here has changed my mind. Having married a master gardener didn't hurt either. It's so gratifying to watch a packet of seeds spring up to become gorgeous flowers or delicious herbs. What a delight to walk outside and snip off a bit of parsley or a few leaves of basil when I'm cooking! You don't need a yard to do this. A few pots on your balcony or windowsill will do. (Another garage sale or thrift store find.) When the herbs get overgrown, just chop some off, put them in baggies, and put them in the freezer. Better yet, share them with your friends and neighbors. They'll love receiving them, and you'll get a warm, fuzzy feeling because you did something nice for somebody else. It can be a lot of pleasure for a very small investment.

Also, learn all you can about your natural surroundings. No matter where you live, there are native flowers, shrubs, trees and grasses. Libraries are full of books to help you. Then when you go out for a walk, you'll be able to recognize and name the things that you see. You'll know the various stages of their growth and look forward to their blooming seasons. You'll feel more a part of the world you live in and be more motivated to walk. And don't discount the value of the Vitamin D you'll be absorbing while being outdoors in the sun.

Food:

I'm not advocating you use food to drown your sorrows, as too many folks tend to do. I'm suggesting that you learn to really appreciate food. Take the time to consciously taste whatever you're eating. Become a connoisseur of those things which are healthy and nutritious, especially vegetables. There are so many ways to prepare vegetables to either enhance or disguise their flavors, depending upon your personal preferences. Grow

123

a few herbs and find some great vegetable recipes that use them. Make each mealtime a really joyous occasion. Use your best dishes, light a candle, and savor each mouthful.

When you're exhausted or in pain or both, the mere thought of cooking a meal can be overwhelming. I only cook on my good days. But, when I do, I make enough for at least two meals. I put the second one in the freezer for the next bad day. Then I can just pop it in the microwave.

Even on a good day, the faster and easier a meal can be put together the better. I've found a great cookbook which helps to do just that. It's called Power Nutrition for your Chronic Illness by Kristine Napier. You'll be amazed at just how quickly and easily you can prepare a really tasty and nutritious meal for yourself and/or for your family.

Afternoon Tea:

Here's one I never would have thought of until I met my second husband. A native Brit, he's rather an expert on the topic. The English have been doing this since Victorian times, and with good reason. "Afternoon Tea" is a lovely tradition with a lot of bang for the buck.

The authentic way is to pour boiling water over loose tea in a ceramic pot, then strain as you pour. However, the same result can be achieved by dropping 3-4 teabags in a 6-cup teapot. It must be black tea, and decaffeinated varieties are available if you need them. Milk is a must, and some like to add a little sugar. Cubes are the most fun. "One lump or two?"

And then there are the scones! If you've never eaten a scone the British way, you're in for a treat. You need two ingredients in addition to the scones. The first is double Devon cream (sometimes called clotted cream). It's a rather pricey delicacy found only in your better supermarkets. However, a little goes a very long way, and it keeps quite a while in the refrigerator. It's well worth the money to make "Having Tea" a really special event. The second thing you need is Lemon Curd. Curd is much less pricey than the cream and is found in most grocery markets next to the jams and jellies.

Begin by breaking or slicing the scone in half horizontally. Spread each half with a layer of double Devon cream, then top with a layer of lemon curd. If you don't have the cream, just use the curd. If you don't have the curd either, use jam. So, there you have it!

Invite some people you know or people you'd like to know better to your home for 4 o'clock tea. That's the official teatime in England. It's a great way to fulfill your social obligations or to repay a kindness with very little fuss or energy. Scones can be made from a mix or purchased in many grocery stores or bakeries. And most people have some tea in their cupboard.

Books:

Today's world is all about TV and videos. Everywhere we look we see ready-made pictures of all the things which were previously left to our own minds to conjure up. Today's technology has robbed us of a simple pleasure unique to each of us: imagination. Don't let this happen to you. Read a book today if you can. I say, "if you can" because I remember a time when I could not.

For many years, I was unable to read a novel. Factual, non-fiction books were manageable. I could somehow get the main ideas. But I could not follow the plot of a novel. Whether I read for 10 minutes or an hour, I couldn't remember where I'd started. Halfway through the book, the characters were still unfamiliar. I have since learned that this inability to read a novel is quite common for people with depression.

It's hard to describe the elation I felt when after many years I was finally able to enjoy a good book again. Since then, I don't take that simple pleasure for granted. Each new book is a treasure to me.

Down pillows:

This is another pleasure that isn't free, but can be a very small price to pay for pain relief. I've suffered from osteoarthritis in my neck and shoulders since my early 20's. Many mornings I couldn't turn my head until I'd been up for several hours. A hot shower was soothing, but the effect only lasted as long as the water did. The buckwheat-filled neck pillows that you heat in the microwave were helpful when first applied but their effect was also only temporary. Trying to go about your day with one of those things tied around your neck is less than comfortable. Aspercream was completely ineffective. Capsaicin burned my skin. Anti-inflammatory drugs irritated my stomach more than they helped my neck. I resigned myself to having constant neck and shoulder pain for the rest of my life - until I discovered down pillows!

Resting my head on a down pillow feels like being cradled by a cloud. I believe the reason it alleviates my neck pain is because it truly gives my muscles an opportunity to relax. A synthetic pillow either has no give at all and holds my head at an abnormal angle, or it has a bounce to it which keeps my muscles tense all night. Whatever the reason, sleeping on a down pillow has resulted in spectacular pain relief for me. I was reminded of exactly how much when I recently slept in a hotel. Although they felt soft to the touch, the pillows in the room were not made of down. My neck affirmed that fact the next morning!

Laughter:

This one is truly free. You can choose to laugh whenever you want to, and it really does relieve pain and depression. Start by stimulating your sense of humor with something you think is really funny. This will be different for everyone. For me, it could be something by Dave Barry or Eddie Izzard. For others it might be a Marx Brothers movie, a 3-Stooges rerun, or an Erma Bombeck classic. Choose something that makes you actually laugh out loud, then buy yourself a copy as your birthday present to you. If you have no current favorites, think of all the fun you'll have experimenting with all the choices available at the library.

And then there's the new craze called Laughter Yoga – although it has little to do with yoga and more to do with stretching, breathing and laughing. Here are two interesting facts that might encourage you to try Laughter Yoga. The first is that your brain doesn't know the difference between real laughter and pretend laughter (i.e. repeating ha-ha-ho-ho-ho). The second is that scientific proof exists that 10 minutes of raucous laughter is the equivalent to 30 minutes of jogging. It releases the same pain-reducing endorphins and improves mood and heart health equally.

After a demonstration held at my monthly FM support group, I experienced a huge decrease in my symptoms – so much so that I searched for a regular laughter club to join. This concept was first developed by an Indian physician named Madan Kataria and was described in his 2002 book called Laugh for no Reason. In his opinion, laughter should be thought of as therapy rather than entertainment and is an excellent cardiovascular exercise. According to Dr. William Fry, one minute of hearty laughter is the cardio equivalent of 10 minutes of jogging.

Laughter Clubs have sprung up all over the world.

Most of them are free. Why not look for one in your area? What have you got to lose?

Whatever your choice, think of laughter as medicine and keep it handy at all times. Use it whenever a downward cycle begins. Don't wait until you're suffering. Be alert to changes in your body, and use your "medicine" as a preventive measure. You might avoid a flare or bring your mood back to normal. The very worst outcome is a few minutes of distraction and relaxation.

Friends:

An old adage says "In order to have a friend, you must be a friend". I couldn't agree more, but I've had to make a slight modification. Lots of days I don't have enough energy to be a friend or much of anything else. But on the days that I do, I try my best to do something nice for someone. I think of it as "giving something to the universe" (Some people call this "paying it forward"). Then when I need something myself, I feel entitled to "take something from the universe". It doesn't matter whether the same person is involved or not. It's all the same to me. I believe that friendship is universal. Perhaps this is just my way of rationalizing having had to accept favors from neighbors and even strangers during particularly difficult times in my life. My theory may be a bit odd, but it works for me. It also helps me to be more "other-person oriented" and less focused on my own troubles and me.

Cuddling:

This makes anybody feel better - young or old, healthy or sick. You don't need to be half of a couple to indulge in this pleasurable pastime. If you live alone, consider a pet. At the very least, get yourself a really cute, really big stuffed animal. Garage sales and thrift stores are great places to find them in new or nearly new condition. No, they don't hug back, but comfort yourself with the fact that you don't need to clean up after them either.

Massage:

I'm not talking about the $75/hr. variety done by a licensed massage therapist, although those are wonderful. You should definitely try one if you can afford it. (See chapter called Touch Therapies.) What I'm talking about is free of charge and can also be effective in blocking pain. It involves only you and your spouse, significant other or very good friend. Begin by warming up some baby oil or body lotion, either in the microwave or by holding the bottle in very hot water. Lay a couple of large towels on top of your bed to soak up any spills, remove as much clothing as you wish, then take turns rubbing each other gently with the oil. Not only does the stroking make sore muscles feel better, it also does wonders for your general well being. If your partner is reluctant to participate because of the fear of hurting you, you go first and demonstrate on him/her how and what you would like done to you.

Candlelight:

This one isn't completely free, but it's very inexpensive. Buy candles when they're on sale in the grocery or drug store, especially after holidays. My table often has red or green candles all year long. Personally, I don't care what color a candle is, lighting a couple of them always makes a table look prettier and makes the food taste better. Even when I lived alone, I lit candles at dinnertime. There's something very soothing to me about watching a flickering flame.

<u>Last, but by no means least, is sex:</u>

This is a difficult issue for many FM people. Although the desire may be present, sex is none too inviting if your FM pain is acting up or if you suffer from a physical limitation. There's nothing remotely sexy about IBS, and depression can rob you of every feeling you ever had. Sexual desire is often the first to go. As a result, many give up the activity altogether.

If, however, you are one of the fortunates who can still enjoy the activity, I highly recommend it. Lisa Stern, a nurse practitioner who works with Planned Parenthood in Los Angeles, says in her blog called Gynfizz.com that the oxytocin released during orgasm triggers endorphins which are responsible for promoting positive emotional states such as bonding and relaxation in addition to pain relief. And, lucky for us, just as our bodies are hypersensitive to pain, they are hypersensitive to pleasure as well. While the pain relief from orgasm is short-lived (usually only 8-10 minutes) past research indicates that even thinking about sex can help alleviate pain. Now, there's a simple pleasure that everyone can enjoy!

There are many additional "Simple Pleasures" that I haven't mentioned here; things like gratitude, helping others and maintaining a positive attitude. The important thing is to be on the lookout for enjoyable pastimes and to experience them whenever you can. The more you're focused on pleasure the less you'll be focused on pain.

Discussion Questions:

> *Have you tried any of these Simple Pleasures?*
> *What results did you have?*
> *What other Simple Pleasures could you add to the list?*

Chapter 18

Take a Deep Breath

B reathing isn't something we normally think about very much. It just happens automatically and keeps us alive. Amazingly, however, the ability to manipulate the breath is also a powerful tool for relaxation and pain control, a pair that go together hand in hand. As with any other skill, the more you practice it, the more proficient you become in using it. In time, the more powerful the effects will be and the longer those effects will last.

Relaxing Breath

My first glimpse into the power of the breath was from Dr. Andrew Weil's wonderful book, Spontaneous Healing. In it he describes his "relaxing breath". Here's how it's done. Inhale to a count of 4. Hold your breath for a count of 7. Exhale audibly for a count of 8. Repeat 5 times. It's that easy. It doesn't matter how quickly or how slowly you breathe in or out. The ratio of 4:7:8 is the important part.

When I first experimented with this exercise, it actually put me to sleep. Now, it just relaxes me, slightly reduces my pain and helps me to gain control of my day. It can be done at any time and in any place. No one will suspect that you're doing it. I often do it in the car when I'm stuck in traffic and would rather be anywhere else or when I'm in an elevator that is stopping at every floor and I'm late for a meeting on the top level.

Foursquare breathing.

Close your eyes and breathe deeply, so that your abdomen expands and contracts like a balloon with each breath. Picture a square. Begin the exercise in the lower left corner. Inhale to a count of four picturing your breath ascending to the top of the square, hold your breath for a count of four, during which time you visualize moving to the right across the top of the box, then exhale to a count of four, picturing descending the right side of the box. Hold for a count of four again while picturing moving back to the left where you began. Repeat for ten cycles. I find this is one of the most distracting breathing techniques available, and I use it often when I find myself in pain and have no other options. It was surprising to me how often the pain completely disappeared, and I needed to take no further measures.

Top to Bottom

Here's one that I often use to prepare for sleep. It's not the same as the familiar relaxation or self-hypnosis technique - the one where they instruct you to first relax the muscles in one place and then do the same in various places as you travel down your body. When I do that one, the result is the opposite of the desired effect. My body gets stiff as a board. You could pick me up with one finger (if you had the strength).

The "Top to Bottom" technique that I do is all about observation. Here it is: First get comfortable. Close your eyes and take a few deep breaths, making the outbreath a bit longer than the inbreath. Practice a few times at first, inhaling as you count to 3, exhaling as you count to 5. It doesn't matter. In a short while, the outbreath will be much longer all by itself.

Next, begin at the top of your head and just observe what it feels like – without trying to change anything or move anything. Feel what your hair feels like where it's attached to your scalp – in the front, above your ears, in the back of your head. Then feel inside of your head. Does one side feel any different from the other? Take another breath in and out, making your outbreath a bit longer than your inbreath. Move your attention down to your forehead. Again, feel what's happening there. Is there tension? Is there pain? If so, does it move around to the back of your head or is it confined to one place? Just observe. Now move down to your eyes, including your eyelids. Continue breathing deeply as you discern what's happening there. Remember, you're not trying to change anything. You're just observing each part of your body as you breathe and relax. Move down to your nose and do the same. Feel the air moving in and out. Feel the outside air on your skin. DO NOT ATTEMPT TO CHANGE ANYTHING! Continue down your entire body until you reach your toes, just taking inventory as you breathe in and more deeply out. Quite often I'm asleep before I get to my knees.

Controlled Deep Breathing

Get into a relaxed position. Either close your eyes or focus on a point. Breathe deeply, using your chest. Think of a 2-syllable word such a "relax" and think it in time with your breathing. Think "peace" on the in breath, think "relax" on the out breath. Repeat for several minutes. This technique is especially helpful to prepare for meditation.

Counting

Whether you count your breaths or count the dimples on your ceiling, one count per breath is a therapeutic technique. Other things you could count are your blessings, your vacations, beautiful views. Anything that takes you away from the here and now will be helpful. The goal here is distraction. Sometimes that's enough to control pain.

The next technique has no name, and I can't remember where I learned it. I just know that it often works for me when I'm having trouble falling asleep. While lying on your back with your eyes closed, take a deep breath in and look up at the ceiling for a few moments, then exhale looking down to the floor. Try not to control when you need the next inhale, just relax and trust your body to do it naturally. Although this is a variation of Jon Kabat-Zinn's Mindfulness Meditation technique which I find difficult to do, I find this modification very simple and relaxing.

Here's another breathing technique that's a form of self-hypnosis. First, lie on your back and close your eyes. In your mind's eye picture the room you're in as being filled with a soft, warm, golden light. This light is called "healing." Everything it touches becomes warm and peaceful and comfortable. Let it touch you. Feel it surrounding your entire body.

Inhale deeply, picturing your breath carrying this golden light from your nostrils inside your body and to the site of your pain. Say to yourself, "In with the healing." Feel it filling the entire painful place. Then exhale more forcefully through your mouth, picturing the pain as darkness exiting your body through your mouth. Think, "Out with the pain." Do this repeatedly, concentrating on bringing the light to each sore spot, one place at a time. Don't be in a hurry.

When you're through, give yourself a few minutes to just lie still and feel the warmth you've created.

Concentrate on the healing that is around you and in you. Then, as you go about your day, continue to picture the healing light within you and the pain leaving your body.

Yoga

The practice of yoga includes many breathing techniques. Several are described in Dennis Lewis's books, Free Your Breath, Free Your Life and The Tao of Natural Breathing. Although he outlines in detail the many benefits of yogic breathing techniques, he also cautions that if done incorrectly, breathing exercises can bring great harm. I would recommend getting some instruction or doing some reading on the topic before using any of these powerful techniques.

You will find many books and internet sites dedicated solely to breathing techniques. My recommendation is to begin slowly and carefully, experimenting with as many as possible after learning as much as you can about each one. You will eventually discover those that will are effective for decreasing some or all of your symptoms.

Consider the breath as one more weapon to include in your arsenal of tools to fight the many facets of fibromyalgia without resorting to a pharmaceutical solution. Healing yourself without drugs yields an unexpected bonus. You'll achieve a feeling of control. That, in itself, is therapeutic.

Discussion Questions:

> *Have you tried breathing techniques?*
> *Where did you learn them?*
> *Which ones work best for you?*

Chapter 19

The Sound of Silence

Whether it's God, The Universe, Yahweh or any other personal deity, a belief in a higher power can bring you comfort when nothing else can. I credit my faith with helping me to cope with many tragedies such as the death of my first husband and the loss of my life as I knew it due to fibromyalgia. I'm grateful for my Catholic upbringing, even though I currently consider myself non-Sectarian. Today I am more spiritual than religious.

Here is a wonderful definition of spirituality written by one of my favorite authors, Brene Brown in her book called The Gifts of Imperfection. "Spirituality is recognizing and celebrating that we are all connected to each other by a power greater than all of us and that our connection to that power and to one another is grounded in love and compassion. Practicing spirituality brings a sense of perspective, meaning and purpose to our lives."

I was raised to believe that prayer was the act of reciting some phrases that I'd memorized from the Baltimore catechism when I was about 7 years old. As a child, all those masses and novenas I attended made me feel quite holy. My private prayers once sounded much like this: "God, help me pass this history test," or "Please, God, let me feel better before I go on vacation next week."

Over the years, my prayers have changed – even though I still do use them. I've learned a thing or two about goals and positive affirmations, mostly from a course I took more than two decades ago called "The Psychology of Achievement" by Brian Tracy. The things I learned in his classes were so powerful and so effective that I still practice them in my own way every day. In fact, I transformed the techniques I learned there into my new form of prayer. There's no doubt in my mind that they played a key role in my ability to recover from my first husband's unexpected death at age 49, the courage to sell my home and move across the country to a place where I knew no one, and the motivation to put my life's experiences into this book.

Note: The Psychology of Achievement course by Brian Tracy is still available from Amazon in CD version. Why not get a set for your car and listen to it or something else of a spiritual nature when you're stuck in traffic and can't do much else?

Getting back to prayer: I now see prayer as a 2-part process. First I talk to God/the Universe/call it what you will. (I call that praying.) Then I give Him/it a chance to talk to me. (I call that meditation.) In my opinion, affirmations are exactly the same as prayers except that they're stated in a positive manner in the present tense. I've also recently added a slight variation – that is to be grateful for something I want even before I receive it. Here's what my prayers sound like today.

I'm grateful that I feel well enough to go out this evening.
I'm grateful that I am loving and kind to everyone I meet.
I'm grateful that I have enough energy to cook dinner.

The key is that each one must be an "I" statement. Anything that follows the words "I am" tells your brain that this is already true for you. Instead of saying, "I won't eat junk food any more, you say, "I'm grateful for eating only healthy food." Instead of "I pray that my book outsells the competition", you say, "I'm grateful that my book is a best-seller."

The more often you repeat these prayers/ affirmations to yourself, the more deeply the ideas get embedded in your brain. Writing them down and then reading them back is even more powerful. But even writing and saying them isn't enough. You must believe that stating what you want is powerful enough to make it happen. And you will! If you repeat your prayers/affirmations over and over <u>with conviction</u>, you will begin to see results, and you will begin to believe in your own power. And, whatever you firmly believe to be true becomes reality for you. It's as simple as that. Well, maybe not quite so simple. People spend their entire lives working at this technique. Personally, it's still new to me, and I'm just beginning to get the hang of it.

There are all kinds of psychological explanations for why this technique works. According to Brian Tracy it's that people attract into their lives the people and circumstances that cause their beliefs to become reality. This is sometimes known as the Law of Attraction. According to believers in the Natural Laws, this one is as powerful as any other natural law, such as the Law of Gravity. Yes, it's all up to us and our brains. And we all know how powerful our brains are. Just think about psychosomatic illnesses, or the placebo effect.

For me, the second part of the prayer process is to listen for advice and/or answers. If your mind is constantly filled with chatter, either from other people, the TV, an iPod or other sources, there is no opportunity for you to hear what God or the Universe or your personal deity has to say to you.

An excellent way to allow this to happen is by meditation. It's a wonderful way to quiet the mind and to become receptive to new knowledge. Totally clearing your mind is nearly impossible to do. However, the process of attempting to do it allows you to notice the thoughts and ideas that refuse to go away. Those are the ones you know you need to address. A quiet mind is fertile ground for new ideas. Those ideas may be exactly what you need to solve your problems, achieve your goals, or answer your prayers.

Meditation is fairly easy to learn; the difficult part is the self-discipline required to incorporate it into your life. It is said that it takes 21 days to develop a habit, so if you can manage 20 minutes a day for this long, you're in! The benefits are endless. If you can take a course to learn how to do it, that's wonderful. If not, read a book or listen to a CD. I've mentioned a few variations here that have been helpful to me, but there are hundreds more to explore.

If this is your first experience with meditation, don't be discouraged if the first method you try doesn't work for you. If it causes you more stress than it relieves, keep looking. But don't give up. Meditation is truly a gift, and one that doesn't cost anything. Search for the technique that brings you peace.

My introduction to meditation was a part of a 3-month course on Stress Management which used Jon Kabat-Zinn's Full Catastrophe Living as its textbook. His technique involves concentrating on the breath without controlling it (easier said than done for a control addict like me). The book is very well written and easy to understand.

An all-day meditation retreat was held at the conclusion of the course. When I first heard about that, I was horrified. The instructor said that previous graduates of the program were invited and that many would probably attend. At the time I thought a person would need to be a little nutty to do this more than once. However, when that day arrived, we meditated from 9 a.m. until 5 p.m.; sometimes sitting, sometimes walking, and sometimes doing yoga, a form of meditation in itself. For the entire day we were not allowed to speak or even to make eye contact with the other attendees (consisting of the 30 people in my class and 36 previous graduates). The effects of that day were profoundly calming and lasted for nearly a week. For those seven days I had very little pain, slept well, and my concentration was better than it had been for a very long time. If I hadn't moved to California, I would have been one of the nutty ones attending the following session's all-day retreat.

Wayne Dyer is another popular author on the topic of meditation. I've read every one of his books, but my personal favorite is Manifest your Destiny which comes with a CD. He teaches his own version of meditation which I find very calming.

But it wasn't until I watched an episode of Dr. Oz when his guest was Deepak Chopra that I learned the form of mediation that I use most often today. It's so simple that I can describe it to you right now.

Assume a comfortable position for you. Close your eyes. Allow your breath to flow in and out effortlessly. Then focus your attention on your heart and ask yourself, "What is my highest vision for my health and well-being?" Let your imagination run wild. What would make you happy? What would that look like and how would it feel? Next, ask yourself, "What is my highest vision for the love and relationships in my life?" Then, "What is my highest vision of my goals for success in life?" And, finally ask "How do I get in touch with my higher self – my spirit? Let all sensations, thoughts and feelings emerge during every step of this process. When you're finished, chant the words, "Ohm bhavam namah" aloud. The rough translation of this Sanskrit phrase is "I am absolute existence: I am a field of infinite possibilities."

Personally, I can't do this process in less than half an hour. During that time I'm focusing on happy, positive things (rather than on how badly I may be feeling), and every time I do it I learn something new about myself. When I'm finished I feel refreshed, relaxed and hopeful. In fact, this practice relaxes me so much that I often fall asleep. When I awaken I finish the rest.

Another form of meditation is called Loving-Kindness Meditation. There are many variations of this one. The easiest one to learn consists of only four sentences that you repeat over and over again. They are:

> May I be filled with lovingkindness.
> May I be free from internal and external danger.
> May I be well in body and mind.
> May I be at ease and be happy.

That's it! Write it down on a 3 x 5 card and pull it out the next time you're feeling low. After you've done it a few times, you won't need the card any more. And you can add more sentences to fill what's missing from your life. But, once again, keep it positive.

Another version of loving-kindness meditation is more outwardly directed and requires a bit more effort Use the same four sentences, but substitute he/she for "I". For example: "May she be filled with lovingkindness". In this exercise, there are four types of persons toward which to direct the lovingkindness. The first is a respected, revered person or a spiritual leader. Next is a family member or friend, then a neutral person (maybe someone who waits on you at Starbucks) and lastly is a hostile person. Start with yourself, then send lovingkindness to each of the above persons. Here's how:

- Visualization: See yourself or the person toward whom you're directing the feeling smiling back at you or just being joyous.
- Reflection: Think of their positive qualities and acts of kindness they have done. Then make a positive statement about yourself.
- Auditory: This is reported to be the most effective. Repeat an internalized mantra or phrase such as "lovingkindness" or "peace and healing" over and over as you breathe deeply..

The purpose of the above (as with all meditations) is to foster positive feelings. When those feelings arise, keep your mind focused on them. If your mind strays, return to the one of the three devices above that aroused them. The second stage is to project those positive feelings outwardly by thinking of loving friends and communities around the world. As your practice matures, it will not be limited to only those you know but will become universal love. Take your good vibrations with you wherever you go, and you will become more friendly and open to everyone you meet.

Note: *For more information on Loving-kindness Meditation, visit www.buddhanet.net.*

The simplest of all the meditations I know was created by Dr. Herbert Benson and is described in the book, Mind Over Medicine by Dr. Lissa Rankin. It's based on transcendental meditation. (Remember that from the 60's?) All that's required is to say a word (a mantra) that resonates with you. It could be "love" or "health" or "ohm" or anything else positive. Breathe slowly and naturally and repeat your word or mantra on the exhale. If thoughts enter your mind, just notice them by saying "Hello worry" or "Hello planning" and gently return to your mantra. This one can even be done with your eyes open while standing, walking, cooking or shopping. Benson recommends doing it for 10-20 minutes twice a day.

Catholics have been saying the Rosary for centuries. When you take a close look, you realize this is another form of meditation. It requires a great deal of focus, and the repetition can be very soothing. It must have worked for my mother. I would often see her sitting on her bed with her beads in her hand. Other religions I know nothing about likely have practices that qualify as meditation as well.

Guided imagery is another powerful technique that is similar to meditation. It focuses the mind and directs the imagination. It may achieve the same results as meditation in that it allows the body to relax and heal itself. Belleruth Naparstek, in her book, Staying Well with Guided Imagery, states that westerners often find this technique easier to use than any other form of meditation because it requires less time and discipline to develop a high level of skill. In addition, appealing sensory images have their own natural pull. The natural trance state it produces can be considered a form of self hypnosis.

Many sources are available if you'd like to give guided imagery a try. There are websites, CD's, podcasts, etc., each one with a different voice. Two websites where you may sample the process of guided imagery before spending any money on a tape, a CD or podcast are www.thehealingmind.org with Dr. Martin Rossman and www.healthjourneys.com with Belleruth Naparstek. Keep in mind that guided imagery is a very personal thing. You may need to explore the individual imagery techniques of several sources before finding one that appeals to you.

To conclude this topic, let me remind you of the story of the drowning man who refuses to be rescued by a man in a boat. "No, thanks," he says, "God will save me." When he later drowns and goes to Heaven, he asks God why He let him drown. And God says, "I didn't let you drown. I sent you a man in a boat, and you refused my help." I believe God (or Yahweh or the Universe, etc.) sends each of us the tools required to deal with the challenges in our lives, including fibromyalgia. We just need to become silent enough to hear them. That's what meditation does.

Discussion Questions:

> *Have you tried meditation?*
> *What form of meditation works for you?*
> *What results do you get when you meditate?*

Chapter 20

Herbal Remedies

At a Fibromyalgia Patient Symposium in Columbus, Ohio many years ago, I spoke with Dr. Mark Pellegrino, a physical medicine doctor, noted fibromyalgia expert and author who suffers from FM himself. I asked him if he had any suggestions for increasing energy. He told me that he'd recently been taking bovine colostrum and that it seemed to be working for him. Given all that he'd accomplished in his life, I considered that to be quite a testimonial.

Bovine colostrum is made from a mother cow's first milk after giving birth. It is reported to be higher in nutrients and lower in fat in order to make it easy for the newborn calf to digest. Although it works for baby cows and Dr. Pellegrino, colostrum didn't work for me.

Supplements, like prescription drugs, produce different results for different people. In addition, they are expensive and not covered by insurance in most cases. Medical schools have not included herbal medicine in their curriculum, so most doctors are of little help in prescribing them or in predicting the effect or interaction they may have with the prescription drugs you're also taking. More importantly, because there are no government standards for supplements, you can't be sure that the bottle contains what it says it does on the label. For this reason, most M.D.'s are reluctant to even recommend them.

To help you sort through all the advertising about supplements as cures for fibromyalgia, I'd recommend you begin by reading a good book on the subject. One that is well researched and easy to understand is Natural Choices for Fibromyalgia written by Jane Oelke, a Naturopathic physician.

I also recommend an online source that tests the various brands of vitamins and supplements on the market. It's called ConsumerLab.com and currently costs $33 a year. Given the amount of money you would waste if you purchased even one untested brand that contained little or none of the substance you thought you were buying, I consider that money well spent.

For years, magnesium with malic acid was one of the first things rheumatologists recommended to their patients diagnosed with FM. It is one of very few natural substances routinely recommended by the medical community. For me, it made no difference in my pain level, but it did produce some improvement in my ability to fall asleep at night. However, it was a "good news", "bad news" situation. The bad news was that I learned that even the smallest amount of oral magnesium gives me the runs. The good news is that with a little research I found that I get all the magnesium my body needs from soaking my feet in Epsom salts (an inexpensive form of magnesium sulfate) for 20 minutes. Just follow the directions on the box. There is also a spray version of magnesium. Initially I tried it on the soles of my feet, purported to be the most absorbent area of the body. That was a mistake. After several applications the skin of my feet peeled off. Now I use it on my wrists and just rub them together. So far, it's working fine.

Often the problem with magnesium is not the

amount you ingest, the problem is with its absorption. If you have IBS with diarrhea, you're likely to be in this category. However, if your tap water is "hard" (meaning it contains high levels of minerals), and you eat whole grains in addition to nuts, fish, and many vegetables, you can usually maintain a normal magnesium level without even taking a supplement. If you're unsure, Dr. Oz claims that four brazil nuts a day will give you all the magnesium you need.

Another widely-accepted natural product is glucosamine. I tried it for an episode of joint pain when it first became popular (I tried it "with chondroitin" and without). After 3 months I concluded that it didn't help me, so I stopped taking it. However, at that time I didn't know that it should be taken along with Vitamin C. (If C bothers your stomach, try ester-C). Years later I tried it again, this time with Ester-C and MSM. The combination worked so well for my ankle, knee and hip pain that I was able to stop taking the prescription drug, Celebrex, and later stopped the glucosamine as well. Now I get along with an occasional Advil when I've been on my feet longer than I should have been.

I had great hope for St. John's Wort when it first hit the market. It has helped many people I know who suffer from depression as I do. One of my General Practitioners who, interestingly, happened to be a Catholic nun, raved about the results she got from it. Because I was unable to tolerate Prozac, Paxil or Zoloft (the only anti-depressants available at the time), I was very keen to try it. Unfortunately, the only effect St. John's Wort had on me was severe diarrhea. This side effect was supposed to go away in time. I persevered for 6 whole days - most of which were spent in the bathroom. Then I gave up.

Sam-e was another disappointment. Two people I knew had experienced almost miraculous improvement in their depression after a few weeks on this supplement. Instead of cheering me up, it made me nauseous.

After becoming disillusioned with supplements, I went to see a nutritionist who was a follower of The Body Ecology Diet, a best-selling book by Donna Gates. After a very detailed and costly consultation, this nutritionist supplied me with a list of "no-no" foods as well as a list of "must-eats." Although I was an adventurous eater, I'd never heard of most of her recommended items. She stressed flax seed oil, rich in Omega-3s, and used it to reduce inflammation. This doesn't taste too bad if you add it to an olive-oil-based salad dressing.

She also recommended raw cultured vegetables to be eaten with every meal to help digestion (Sauerkraut is an acceptable substitute). As vile as the taste was, my reflux and my IBS improved greatly. There was also a liquidy form of yogurt called kefir, which was to be drunk instead of eating a meal. Kefir is an excellent source of acidophilus which are some of the good bacteria in your colon. It is also helpful for IBS.

The drinks she suggested were worse than the foods. Apple cider vinegar mixed with water and sipped throughout the day was supposed to quell the urge to consume anything that tasted good and was therefore verboten. There were different teas for every symptom. They all tasted terrible, but by far the worst was made from a form of dried seaweed called Kombu. Try as I might, I just couldn't swallow that oily stuff after the first sip. And I really tried. It was reputed to be wonderful for depression, and that was my worst problem at the time.

If you're prone to digestive problems like IBS and/or GERD (gastro-esophageal reflux disease), a nutritionist's advice can be especially valuable. For example, did you know that a single slice of radish soaked in Umeboshi vinegar greatly improves the digestion of a protein meal? That was a tip from my nutritionist. If you can remember to cut up a radish and keep it soaked and store it in the refrigerator, it really does work!

The food-form vitamins she recommended made perfect sense to me. If they were made from food, how could they be bad for you? She also recommended a powdered substance reputed to contain the trace minerals that have been depleted from our soil and therefore missing in the vegetables we eat. Unfortunately, the vitamins and the powder were only available by mail order from a company with which this nutritionist was associated. After my initial $120 purchase, I was invited to also become a representative of the company in some sort of a pyramid marketing arrangement. I declined.

I don't mean to give nutritionists a bad name. They do important work, and they're not all trying to sell you something. It's just that most people (including me) are so accustomed to eating the wrong foods that the recommended dietary changes seem positively radical and most taste quite radical as well.

Nutritionists routinely recommend taking a probiotic which is live bacteria that may confer a health benefit on the host. When a person takes an antibiotic, for example, the good bacteria as well as the harmful ones are affected, sometimes causing unpleasant symptoms.

When considering the purchase of a probiotic, keep in mind the four criteria used to rate them: their culture count (at least 15 billion is recommended), the number of strains (at least 10, more is better, each starting with L for lacto or B for bifido), their potency at expiration (rather than when they were put in the bottle) and whether or not they have delayed release (meaning they remain in the stomach long enough to compete with the acidity there).

VSL#3 is one of the few probiotic preparations supported by double-blind, placebo-controlled scientific studies (one of which was published in the July 2005 edition of the American Journal of Gastroenterology). Each capsule contains 112.5 billion live bacteria. Whether it's the best or merely the most examined won't be known until and unless further studies are done.

Supplements are used extensively in the alternative form of medicine called Ayurveda. I wandered into this world quite by accident. A chiropractor I visited for my neck pain incorporated this ancient Indian self-care practice into his treatments. Again there were supplements to purchase, but none of them tasted awful, and a few were even quite helpful. One was the herb, Boswellin, used for joint pain. It was so effective that I was able to reduce by half the amount of anti-inflammatory medication I was taking at the time. After several months, I stopped taking both of them completely. Even ten years later, I rarely have ankle, knee or hip pain.

These days whenever a new symptom appears I consult "The" book on Ayurveda called Perfect Health by Deepak Chopra. He is the guru of the subject whom you may have seen on several talk shows. Because the tenets of Ayurveda are so benign, I usually follow them first. If there's no improvement, then I go to see my doctor. In my opinion, Ayurveda is beneficial for anyone and particularly helpful for those with fibromyalgia. I would caution you, however, about taking Ayurvedic preparations imported from India. There have been instances of heavy metal poisoning reported. This would be another instance when membership in Consumer Labs would be helpful. It would assist you in deciding which brand of a particular herb is worth the money.

Another herbal treatment fibro people often pursue is aromatherapy. Although herbs can be powerful healers, they can also be surprisingly dangerous. What we don't know can indeed hurt us, and this is an area about which the layperson knows very, very little. Because so many FM people suffer from Multiple Chemical Sensitivity, I'm hesitant to recommend aromatherapy. However, I feel I must share with you some important things I learned from a course I took from a biologist and experienced herb grower and essential oil producer.

Essential oils are not oils at all. They are concentrated extracts of plants, distilled either by steam or by pressing. In order to use them for massage, a diluting agent or carrier oil such as grape seed must be used. Use no more than 12-18 drops of essential oil to an ounce of carrier oil. Never apply undiluted essential oils to your skin. Before using an essential oil as a massage, test a drop of the diluted oil on the inside of your wrist or elbow. Cover it with a cotton ball and a band-aid and leave it for 24 hours. If there's any reaction, do not use it.

To use an essential oil in a vaporizer, use 2 drops of the essential oil in a glass atomizer full of water. Spray once or twice into the room. To use it in a diffuser, put a couple of drops of oil on the unglazed portion of a terra cotta device, cap it and leave it on a table or desk. An alternative solution is to place a few drops on a cold light bulb.

Each essential oil has unique characteristics. For example, peppermint oil opens the sinuses and stimulates conversation. A couple of diffusers in a room are good when you invite a group of people for a party. Ylang-ylang is an anti-depressant. Lavender is calming. The list goes on and on.

Because scents can access areas of the brain that nothing else can touch, essential oils can be powerful healers. They can also be toxic. Never swallow an essential oil. Wintergreen oil, for one, can be fatal if ingested. Even if properly diluted, essential oils should never be used regularly for more than 3 weeks. A systemic build-up can occur.

Be sure that any oil you purchase is all natural. The scent of a synthetic oil can give you an instant headache or nausea. In fact, that could be a tip-off that it's not a true essential oil. There are no health benefits from synthetic oils.

Purchase only oils which are clear or just slightly tinted. If they're dark or thick, they're old or have been opened. Manufactured products that claim to contain essential oils have had the active ingredient removed in the processing. For example, the active ingredient of thymol has been removed from the essential thyme oil purported to be in some toothpastes.

If you're considering using essential oils, learn all you can about them before you do. Be aware that they are very powerful - both for healing and for harming. Be particularly careful if you have allergies or sensitive skin. Extreme caution should be taken if you have high blood pressure, a chronic illness, or are pregnant. An excellent book on the subject is Aromatherapy for Everyone by PJ Pierson and Mary Shipley.

A website that lists many of the oils and their uses is http://www.family-essential-oils.com/essential-oil-use-chart.html. Remember that for topical application, an essential oil must always be diluted with a carrier oil. This site has information on that process as well. Be sure to read and follow their directions.

If you're considering using an herbal remedy of any kind, I recommend you seek out a reputable health food store and establish a relationship with an educated staff member. Be sure to tell him/her what prescription drugs you're taking. He will be able to suggest an appropriate supplement for a specific ailment. More importantly, he will know if a companion product is necessary to improve its absorption in the body. He will also know what brands are more effective, how much to take, and how long before you should see a result. You may pay a bit more for supplements at a health food store, but you're paying for their knowledge in addition to the product. As a result, it could end up costing you less money in the long run. Additionally, a health food store is often willing to refund your money if an item they recommended doesn't work for you.

Years of research, experimentation, and expense have proven to me how unique each human body is. If you wish to try supplements, here is my advice: Check with your doctor before ingesting anything new. Supplements can and do cause dangerous interactions with prescription drugs. Even though medical doctors are often unfamiliar with herbal supplements, they may be quite aware if a particular one interacts with a drug he's prescribing for you.

If your physician is unable to advise you or you become overwhelmed with supplements that don't seem to be working, consider a visit to a naturopathic physician. This is something that I have done recently with wonderful results. It took me a long time to take this step because naturopathic services are not covered by insurance in California. However, in Connecticut, all insurance companies cover naturopaths. It's just a matter of time before the rest of the states fall in line. Just look at what has happened with chiropractic services, acupuncture and massage therapy.

A word of caution:

Beware of unscrupulous people trying to sell you something/anything. It is well known that people with

155

fibromyalgia become discouraged with ineffective medical therapies and are looking for nonconventional answers to their problems. People will try to sell us just about anything - from tonics to orthotics - and call it a "cure" for fibromyalgia.

Discussion Questions:

> *What supplements have you tried and what were your results?*
> *How do you judge whether a supplement brand is reliable or not?*
> *Where did you learn about supplements that have helped you?*

Chapter 21

Pot or Not

No discussion of herbal remedies would be complete without the inclusion of cannabis, politely known as medical marijuana. If it's not legal in your state, please proceed to Chapter 20 – until the Federal Government admits its error in classifying marijuana as a Class 1 drug "with no currently accepted medical use" and approves usage by all. Many FM sufferers are either ignorant or fearful of its effects. For a long time I was one of them. For that reason, I share my experience with you.

I somehow survived college in the 60's without ever having smoked a marijuana cigarette. It's not that I was opposed on moral or legal grounds. It's just that I could never get the smell past my nose. My chemical sensitivities were in overdrive, even then. I still find the odor hugely offensive.

So now there I was, a bona fide, card-carrying AARP member and a marijuana virgin. A physician who spoke to our FM support group gave me the courage to finally try it. A Board Certified Family Practitioner and former cannabis researcher at UCLA, he is the source of everything I know about this herb. When compared to all the information that's available, it's precious little.

Basically, two of the three varieties of cannabis are used for medical purposes. They are indica and sativa. Indica tends to be a downer and sativa tends to be an upper. Both varieties contain as many as 64 cannabinoids. The two most commonly known are: tetrahydrocannabinol (aka THC), the portion that elevates your mood) and cannabidiol (aka CBD), the portion that calms anxiety and reduces pain. CBD has no psychotropic effects by itself but reduces the higher anxiety levels produced by THC alone. The higher the CBD to THC ratio, the more effective its pain-relieving ability.

There are several synthetic cannabis medications approved by the FDA in the US as well as two that actually contain the cannabis herb. Because herbs are not patentable, the drugs available in the U.S. contain only one of the two essential elements of cannabis rather than both. Unfortunately, the entire herb is required for the desired effect. As a result, these drugs have side effects similar to other pain-relieving medications. In the UK, Canada and most European countries, a spray called Sativex is available that does contain the entire herb and is currently available by prescription for the treatment of multiple sclerosis. It will soon be approved for cancer pain and neuropathic conditions as well.

Although marijuana is now legal for recreational use as well as for medical use in California, the sad truth is that the process is far from user friendly. Very few physicians want to be associated with cannabis use, so this means finding a doctor you don't know whose entire practice likely consists of evaluating patients for marijuana use. The term "evaluate" means quickly scanning some paperwork you brought with you containing your diagnosis, taking a blood pressure reading, and signing a form. This doc is often employed by a non-profit organization and works out of a dilapidated office with dirty walls and stained carpeting and a waiting room interspersed with tattooed teens whose only medical problem is that they drank too much the night before.

Once a recommendation is obtained, the real challenges begin. The first is to purchase your product, legally available only from a dispensary or a collective. Apparently nobody wants one of these places in their neighborhood. As a result, they are located in the seediest sections of town. Prohibited from advertising in any way, their only signage is just some initials above the door.

Upon entering a dispensary, you present your official card and driver's license to a bouncer, then walk through a screening device similar to those used at the airport. After that your credentials are verified. Then and only then are you escorted to the inner sanctum where the products are for sale.

Armed with my new-found knowledge, my goal was an herb with a high CBD to THC ratio. What I found was a whole new world consisting of hundreds of hairy-looking objects inside glass jars, each clearly labeled with names that commonly included the words "kush" or "haze", each one a hybrid with no indication of CBD or THC content. I was at the mercy of a clerk who may or may not have known anything about the products for sale. After purchasing my 1/8 oz. of "grass" for $32, I hurried outside, more than a little concerned that my car might have been vandalized by the unseemly-looking characters loitering across the street when I arrived. The whole experience left me feeling a bit scummy and anxious to go home and take a bath.

The next decision was how to ingest the stuff. Although the doctor's advice was a spray tincture to apply under the tongue, I couldn't find it for sale anywhere in the Los Angeles area. His second choice was a vaporizer, so I decided I would purchase one of those. The advantage of vaporizing over smoking is that the machine only heats the weed to a temperature where it gives off its oils in the form of steam, thereby eliminating harmful poisons created by the burning process and drastically reducing the smell. Unfortunately, the places that sell the product often don't sell the equipment needed to use the product.

I next visited a local "head shop" hoping to get some much-needed advice from the people working there. Unfortunately, the multi-pierced clerk used mostly slang terms I didn't understand. Too embarrassed to ask for clarification when I didn't even understand the lingo, I purchased the most expensive selection along with the required grinder for a grand total of $300, grabbed the instructions, and left in a hurry.

Upon arriving home, I realized that the instructions that come with a vaporizer only tell you how to assemble the machine. Apparently, the assumption is that you know how much weed to use, how finely to grind it, how to pack it in the device as well as how strongly to inhale it, as well as how many inhales it takes to get the desired effect – that being pain relief rather than unconsciousness. To say there's a steep learning curve involved with marijuana use is an understatement.

What I needed was an experienced user. I finally found a friend of a friend who grew his own and vaporized daily for back pain relief. He was willing to instruct me in its use and sell me some he had grown. We used his vaporizer and his weed. He went first, took one deep drag, then handed the tube to me. I did the same, employing the deep yoga breathing technique I thought was necessary. After one inhale, he suggested waiting 15 minutes to see what the effect might be. I began to feel light headed, then a little giddy, and then I just got happy. It was the happiest I'd ever felt in my life, and it lasted for 6 hours. I was in love with life!

Determined to repeat the process frequently, I purchased some weed from him and left. Unfortunately, he moved away a short time later and I was left to fend for myself. Now I had to duplicate the experience at home on my own.

The effort of putting the contraption together, waiting for it to heat up, standing there while it achieved the required temperature and the anxiety of wondering whether I'd inhale too much or not enough was more aggravation than I cared to endure, especially at 3 a.m. when I was desperate for sleep.

There were a few times when marijuana did put me right to sleep – a wonderful outcome for an insomniac like me. But there were other times when I saw disturbing sights when I closed my eyes. Even though I knew the source, I still felt total panic. It wasn't anything I'd care to do again, but I don't wish to discourage anyone else from trying it. One woman in my FM support group smokes it on a daily basis – one inhale before work, one upon arriving home. She claims it keeps her pain under control so she can work and keeps her mind functioning as well. Unfortunately she grows only the amount she uses and has no idea which variety it is, so she was no assistance in my education.

Perhaps now that it has become mainstream, marijuana education will be more available, the products will become more standardized, and its use will become as common as aspirin. I'm confident that a day will come when the consumer will know exactly what strain and how much to purchase, exactly how to ingest it for best results and what those results may be.

I'm even hopeful that one day the conservative conventional medical community will embrace its use. Until that happens, count me out.

Discussion Questions:

Have you used cannabis to treat your FM symptoms?
Was it helpful?
Describe your experience.
How did you learn to use it?

Chapter 22

Touch Therapies

At a Fibromyalgia Symposium I attended several years ago I was introduced to a woman who is a born healer. I've never met anyone like her before or since. Her voice, her touch, her caring manner affected me so greatly that I allowed her to use me as a guinea pig in a demonstration she was giving on the art of reflexology (sometimes known as acupressure). Because I'm a terrible skeptic, I must admit to having had very little faith in this practice before it was done to me. However, without knowing anything about my history or my symptoms, this reflexologist picked up my feet and, using only her thumb, she pressed on a few places until she found a horribly painful spot. Holding her thumb there, she instructed me to breathe deeply and relax as she held the pressure. In a few short seconds the pain I'd been feeling in my knees was completely gone and was replaced by a soothing warmth. Although I hadn't mentioned it to her, my knees had been sore and swollen from over-activity that day when she began. Claiming the pain had been due to blocked energy, she pressed on the same spot on my foot again. This time there was no pain at all. Better yet, the pain in my knees was still gone as well.

After her initial success, I began to tell her where

the other painful areas were on my body. She then skillfully moved her thumbs to the correspondingly painful places on my feet. Each time, after one short stab of discomfort during which I was instructed to relax and breathe deeply, each pain was replaced by a comforting warmth, and I was pain free. My entire body began to relax. When she was finished I felt completely peaceful and comfortable for the first time in many months. I slept more soundly that night than I had in years and continued to be pain free the next morning.

I would later learn that my reflexologist had been Linda Chollar, one of the premier touch practitioners in the United States. In addition to being a board accredited Reflexology Educator, she is a State licensed massage therapy instructor. She is also certified in polarity therapy, cranial-sacral therapy and Reiki. For more than twenty years she has taught at massage schools, hospitals, nursing schools, and maintains a private practice in Redondo Beach, Ca. as well. Linda can be reached at www.PainFreePath.com.

Linda and I later became friends, and she explained to me how reflexology works. Practitioners work from maps. Each nerve in our body ends in the feet. The result is a miniature image (or map) of the entire body, each foot representing a vertical half. For example, the liver is on the right side of the body, and therefore the corresponding reflex area is on the right foot. There are similar maps on the hands and the ears. What most people don't understand is that reflexology is not designed to diagnose or cure illness. Rather, its function is to relieve discomfort which allows the body to heal itself.

Do not mistake a strip mall reflexology spa with treatment from a certified reflexologist. The difference is similar to that between treatment from a masseuse and a massage therapist. Education is the key. However, in my experience, a masseuse with little knowledge of the body can actually cause you serious pain, an untrained reflexologist would likely have no effect at all – unless you enjoy having your feet manipulated for half an hour. Just don't expect any decrease in your symptoms.

I made the mistake of going to a highly-recommended masseuse who was skilled in relieving sore muscles of active athletes but knew nothing about fibromyalgia. She dug her fingers deep into the knots in each of my sore muscles. At the time she was doing it, it felt really good. By that evening I began to feel sore. The next day I could barely get out of bed, and I hobbled around in extreme pain for the next several days. This was a case of too much too soon.

What massage does is to circulate the lactic acid that accumulates in your joints. That's often the source of pain. However, when too much lactic acid gets dumped into your system at one time, the results can be disastrous, especially for sensitive people like those of us with FM. When done by a knowledgeable massage therapist, it can be a wonderful therapy. I suggest asking your physician or another FM patient for a referral if you're interested in trying it.

A lot of people shy away from chiropractors, and I can understand why. I've been to a few I wouldn't recommend to anyone. A couple were very rough. Each adjustment felt like my bones were breaking. Many sell nutritional supplements to augment their income, and they ardently promote a purchase at every visit. Others advertise themselves as "fibromyalgia specialists" and sell pricey multi-month packages of treatments that must be paid for in advance. I would check with the Better Business Bureau before contracting with any of them.

In general, experience has taught me that most chiropractors don't know enough about fibromyalgia to be of much help. But I was desperate. I could feel that my spine was crooked. As a result, I was suffering from acute nerve pain that required opiates as often as 3 times a week. So I took a chance. I didn't have high expectations for his ability to help me. However, his office was one of the few that accepted my insurance, it was located close to my home, so I went. Thanks to this dedicated healer and his gentle ministrations, I haven't needed opiates for many months. Rather than try to sell me on more adjustments as many chiropractors do, his goal was to strengthen the muscles next to my spine to hold his adjustments in place. The desired result was to reduce the number of visits I needed to make to his office. He prescribed exercise to help with this and supervised every step of the process to ensure that his staff of physical therapists were treating my tender body differently than they treated the robust athletes who were their usual clients. I still receive the occasional adjustment when I feel myself getting crooked or when I've overdone some physical activity.

Recently, I've discovered a device called a foam roller. It's about 6" in diameter, 18" long, made from a sturdy material covered with soft foam. The technique is to lay on the floor, place the roller under your neck, lock your fingers behind your head, then roll backwards. (Be sure to wear shoes with gripping soles if you're doing this on a carpeted floor). I was amazed to hear the same popping, cracking noises I thought only chiropractors could coax from my back. Because I'm a back sleeper, I can feel when my back is even the slightest bit out of place. One roll on my foam roller after a few minutes on a heating pad, and it's often all better. My physical medicine doctor recently cautioned me against using this therapy too often.

When overdone (like most other things) long-term negative effects can and do occur. But, for me, it's made a huge difference. If nothing else, it's given me a sense of control I never had before. That, in itself, is huge. But, more importantly, this device has successfully prevented some excruciating muscle spasms that once caused me to be a regular visitor to the local Emergency Room.

Physical therapy can also be helpful to FM patients. If pain or fatigue is preventing you from participating in a particular activity, gentle manipulations can be done as well as demonstrations of stretching and exercise techniques for you to do at home. I found it very helpful when I was having extreme difficulty climbing stairs due to shaky muscles in my legs. Again, insurance coverage might be an issue. Be sure to check your policy. You might need to be referred by a specialist.

Acupuncture has become mainstream and is covered by more and more insurance policies. As with all professionals, some are more knowledgeable than others. Or, perhaps, they are more experienced in dealing with FM symptoms. I had three completely ineffective treatments before finding an acupuncturist who is really skilled.

When we first met, I was suffering from withdrawal symptoms. No, I wasn't an addict. Rather I was abruptly taken off a benzodiazepine by a psychiatrist who should have known better. Not realizing the potential for disaster, I followed her instructions. The result was the kind of withdrawal you see in horror movies. I trembled. I shook. I was anxious and depressed. I couldn't concentrate. I couldn't function. I lost 25 lbs. in 2 months. It was the worst experience of my life. Conventional medicine could only prescribe more drugs which I was afraid to take. When I finally did, they provided little help.

Then a friend referred me to an acupuncturist who had experience treating withdrawal symptoms. She literally saved my life. At first I saw her 3 times a week. Two years later I still receive treatments, but now it's only once every 2 or 3 weeks – for a "tune-up" as she calls it.

In case you're wondering, there is very little or no pain at all when a skillful acupuncturist inserts her needles. Each one is about the size of a human hair. Following the principles of Chinese medicine, acupuncture is based on the energy meridians in the body – similar to reflexology. Theoretically, when they are blocked, you have problems. The job of the acupuncturist is to unblock them. Sometimes it can be done in a single visit. Other times several visits are required. If you're doubtful about the effectiveness of acupuncture, keep in mind that it's used as anesthesia for major surgery in China.

If acupuncture is not in your budget, you might consider self-acupressure. It's based on the same system of meridians that acupuncture and reflexology are, but it's done with finger pressure instead of needles. With a larger area to work with (your fingertip versus a tiny needle) you may still be able to obtain benefit from gentle pressure in the general location. Stimulation of these places is said to release endorphins, the natural pain-relieving substance in the body. A map of the body's meridians should be available from a book at your local library.

Ayurveda also has a touch therapy that I have found effective. The practice is called abhyanga. It's been popularized by Deepak Chopra and Dr. Andrew Weil among others. Abyanga involves massaging your own body with refined sesame oil, the kind sold in health food stores. After warming it a little, you begin with the soles of your feet and massage about a teaspoonful into each one. Then you move to the head and work your way downward, applying the oil in a circular motion on your scalp and torso, using long, quick strokes on your arms and legs. Done before a shower, it's not as messy as it sounds. You should allow a few minutes for it to penetrate, during which time you can brush your teeth, tweeze your eyebrows, etc. Not only does abhyanga feel good, but it does wonders for dry skin as well. I find this especially comforting during flares. Done regularly, it may even help to prevent them.

The common goal of any touch therapy is to induce a relaxation response that helps the body to heal itself. I suggest you try one of more of them to see if they make a difference for you. Be aware that few of them (with the exception of some chiropractic and some massage therapy) are covered by insurance. Always inquire about their rates in advance. And keep pushing your insurance company to cover alternative treatments. They are useful adjuncts to conventional medicine, especially for people with chronic illnesses like FM and, in particular, for those of us who have difficulty with side effects from conventional medications. If you find a therapy that works for you, chances are you'll need less medication and be able to participate more fully in life. In the long run, insurance companies would save themselves money if they covered these therapies. The problem is that they are yet to be convinced.

Discussion Questions:

> *What was your best or worst experience with a touch therapy?*
> *Which one (if any) would you recommend and why?*

Chapter 23

Write it Down

Perhaps the best advice I have for anyone suffering from fibromyalgia is Document Everything. You never know when you'll need it, and you'll learn more about yourself than you ever dreamed possible. You and your doctor will rely on this information to help you cope with your fibromyalgia symptoms.

The easiest record to keep is a daily diary. You don't need to write complete sentences. You don't need a lot of words. Just get yourself a small spiral notebook and keep it next to your bed. Before you go to sleep, write down what kind of day you had. Include things like the items listed below and anything else you consider pertinent – just a few words to jog your memory.

You'll want to keep two kinds of information; medical and non-medical. Unless you write it down, it's gone. I once was known for my excellent memory. But it's gone now - lost in fibrofog someplace.

The Medical Stuff:

How You Feel. This is important for so many reasons. If you write down other things as well, you will begin to see when and why you feel the way you do. You'll know how various foods, medications or activities affect you. For example, you'll want to remember that the day after you walked half a mile your knees swelled up and you couldn't drive a car. The next time it's necessary for you to drive somewhere, you won't make the mistake of walking a long distance the day before.

Medications: Write down everything you took that day - what it was, (if a generic, note the manufacturer) how much you took, and when you took it. Then you'll know if it's better to take a particular drug or supplement with a meal or on an empty stomach or if it doesn't make a difference. When listed with the other data on your list, you'll be able to compare the way you feel now with the way you felt before taking the drug so you'll know whether it had any effect at all.

Most important of all: Write down any and all side effects you might have had from taking the medication. Approximately 10 years ago, it became apparent that I was a paradoxical responder. What that means is that if the warning on the label said "may cause drowsiness", I knew I'd be up all night. If the warning said "may cause constipation", there was a good chance I'd be unable to leave the house the next day due to diarrhea. Since then I have kept a list of all the drugs that gave me side effects, the dosage I took and the side effects they caused. The list is with me at all times. Some physicians are intimidated by my list. Others are grateful to know what I'm able to tolerate. Me, I just want to save myself unnecessary misery. At last count, there were 97 drugs on my "Side Effects" list. I also keep a list of drugs that were well tolerated. Unfortunately, that's a much shorter list.

Symptoms and their Severity:

Rank your symptoms on a scale of 1 to 10 (10 being the worst). Include pain, fatigue, cognitive ability, IBS, TMJ (temporomandibular joint disorder), insomnia or anything else that plagues you regularly. If you ever need to prove disability, a record of your daily symptoms is invaluable. Fibromyalgia doesn't go away, and you can't remember everything forever.

Doctor Encounters:

It's a good idea to take your journal with you when you visit your doctor - or at least read it over before you go, and jot down a few of the key medical issues you've been dealing with since your last visit. Try to limit your list to the three most troublesome problems. There's just so much that can be discussed in a single appointment and just so much advice you can absorb.

During or immediately after your visit, make a note of any new suggestions, medications, etc. that you were given. It's so much easier to record it when it's fresh in your mind than to try to remember it several days later. It's also a good idea to bring a friend or loved one with you to your appointment. Even if you take copious notes as I do, it's always helpful to have another set of ears and another memory to rely upon.

If you want to go the extra mile (which you may want to do if you're having a particularly difficult time dealing with your symptoms) download the FM Daily Symptom Form found on my website @ www.fmspubs.com. This form will help you to convey how you're feeling to your doctor. I created it by using one that was designed by a physician for his patients with FM and making modifications I felt were necessary. Many fellow patients have found it to be useful as well.

I also keep a card in my wallet with all my doctors' names, their specialties, addresses and phone numbers. This is handy for making appointments and filling out insurance forms or when I forget where a particular doctors office is located or if I need to call from my car to say I'll be late. My pharmacy phone number is also on the list. It's handy in case a prescription needs to be phoned in. If you're an avid cell phone user, this information could be recorded there instead.

The Non-Medical Stuff:

Activity. If you went to the grocery store, write it down. If you met a friend for lunch or took a long walk, write it down. You'll be surprised to learn how each activity affects you. This you will know by reading your entries for the next day or two.

Sleep. If you only slept 3 hours during the night, write it down. If you got through the day without a nap, write it down. You'll learn how important sleep is to your quality of life. I find that lack of sleep makes my cognitive ability much worse than normal and also increases my pain level.

Weather. If the sun's been shining for 5 consecutive days, write it down. If it's been raining for 24 hours, write it down. Then notice how you feel that day and the next day. A changing barometer affects most fibromites, including me. Whether it denotes a change for the better or for the worse makes no difference. Any change affects the way I feel. When the sun is shining, I feel much better than I do on a dreary day. If the weather is dry, I feel much better than I do when it's humid. If you find that you do, too, then you might want to rethink a vacation to London or Seattle in favor of one to Phoenix or Albuquerque.

Food. Yes, write down what you ate and drank, especially if it was unusual or a change from what you normally eat or drink - either in content or quantity. You might see a correlation between what you ingest one day and how you feel the next day. For example, I learned that more than one glass of wine with dinner often gives me heart palpitations the next day. I also learned that eating a chocolate dessert after dinner keeps me awake at night.

To give you an idea of what may be helpful to write down, here are a few of my own journal entries. (The numbers in parentheses indicate severity)

1/2/05 Warm day. Had company for tea outside this afternoon. No nap. Too much sugar. Pain (8) in neck and shoulders (7). Exhaustion (10) by 8 p.m. Went to bed. Too much pain to sleep.

1/3/05 Awoke with headache (5). Drank black tea, helped a little. Short walk with dog. Saw Dr. after waiting 2 hours in his waiting room. Felt angry and resentful. Will seek new rheumatologist. Will reduce Flexeril to 7.5 mg. and try swimming again.

1/4/05 Only slept 2 hours last nite. Gas pains and diarrhea in a.m. Short walk. Very windy. Slept 3 hours in p.m. Awoke depressed. Too exhausted (9) to cook dinner. Ordered pizza.

1/5/05 Couldn't sleep again. Finally took Ambien at 2 a.m. Slept till 9. Felt better today. Swam at Y in a.m., then did laundry. Napped 2 hours. Sunny day. Mood better.

Now you get the idea. Once you get in the habit (A habit usually takes 21 days to create.) it only takes a couple of minutes. The more information you have the better you'll be able to control your symptoms and to help yourself feel better.

Last, but not least, USE WHAT YOU LEARN!!! It does no good to discover that eating too much sugar increases your pain and fatigue if you continue to eat too much sugar. If a new symptom pops up, review your last few journal entries. You may discover exactly what is causing it. If not, keep writing. Eventually it may become clear. Perhaps you'll save yourself a doctor visit. If not, you'll attend with enough information that the two of you will be better prepared to figure it out together.

Discussion Questions:

> *What medical records do you keep for yourself?*
> *Do you find the answers you need when you need them?*
> *What information do you wish you had kept?*

Chapter 24

Support Groups
Are Not Created Equal

B e aware that support groups vary greatly. The best ones are often sponsored by a hospital. The staff often assists with the administration, and they have access to speakers who will be available to attend meetings and to provide pertinent and useful information. Next to your doctor, it's the best place to get your questions answered. For most people, it's their only opportunity to meet people who truly understand their problems.

The way FM impacts each life varies from person to person. For this reason, one specific group will not be the right fit for all. However, there are some general characteristics to keep in mind when deciding whether to join any particular group.

The good groups keep you informed and offer true support. Others can be nothing more than gripe sessions. Attending one of these meetings can leave you feeling drained and hopeless. The common cause is usually lack of leadership. Folks who have the illness themselves often lead these groups out of necessity. No one else is willing to do it. This, in itself, is not a bad thing. However, the quality of the programming and the group's very existence are determined by the leader or leaders' current state of health. I know. I have led such a group myself. The most important thing I learned from my experience is the importance of having a co-leader. Chances are, both of you won't be having a flare at the same time.

If you've never participated in a support group, you're probably wondering what joining a group can do for you. There are two main benefits. The first involves people. The second involves education.

People:

- Support groups give you an opportunity to interact with people like you – people whose lives are impacted by illness on a daily basis. Yes, it's true! Misery does love company. Living in a world mostly populated by healthy people can be very lonely for someone with a chronic illness. Old friends tend to drift away after numerous cancellations due to a sudden emergence of symptoms, but new friendships form easily with people who live with the same challenges you face each day.

- Attending a meeting can be a reason to get out of the house and go to a place where nothing is expected of you (except to be kind to the other members). It's a place where you will be accepted – problems and all.

- People naturally bond together to fight for common goals – whether it's improved quality of life for each group member or issues such as increased awareness for fibromyalgia, funding for FM research, or increased benefits from health or disability policies. Focusing on any of these things is healthier than focusing on your own symptoms.

- My personal feeling is that a support group is successful to the degree it instills a feeling of "family" in the group. When helping each other becomes the central focus, the group truly provides "support".

Education:

- Learn how other people cope with the same situations you face each day.
- Learn about new products that are available to help you feel better or make your life easier.
- Learn results of new research to discuss with your doctor and incorporate into your own treatment plan.

LOCATE AN EXISTING SUPPORT GROUP

Here are some suggestions for finding a group that already exists where you live.

- www.fmcpaware.org provides a geographic listing.
- The American Chronic Pain Assn. has an online list of groups by state.
- The Pro Health website (www.prohealth.com) has a support group finder where you can search by city, state or ailment. They also have a chat room you can join.
- The Arthritis Foundation sponsors groups in many areas and may be willing to help you start a group of your own. They also train support group leaders. Contact them at www.arthritis.org.

- Check with your own doctor as well as with other general practice and rheumatology offices in your area.
- Call area hospitals, the library, local newspapers, radio and TV stations.
- Some groups may not have fibromyalgia in their name, but they will welcome you just the same. The name may indicate that a particular group is for fibromyalgia, chronic fatigue, chronic pain, chronic illness, arthritis or something similar. Most groups are open to anyone with a related illness. If you have any doubts, call the contact person and ask. If that group is not for you, he/she may know of another group that is.

Chapter 25

Forming a Fibromyalgia Support Group

When no fibromyalgia support group exists in your local area, consider forming a group of your own. It's not all that difficult, but it does take some time and effort. If you can enlist the help of another fibromyalgia patient, the process will become a lot easier and faster. Chances are, you will also make a friend for life.

It's helpful to discuss your intentions with your fibro-friendly doctor. Ask if you can count on his support. He may know someone at the local hospital who might be willing to assist you. At the very least, get his permission to post a notice in his waiting room to announce the formation of your group.

The next order of business is to find a place to hold an organizational meeting. You could call your local hospital and ask about meeting rooms there. Or you can ask at the local library. Banks and churches offer their meeting rooms for community groups as well.

Make a list of times available at each location. This way you can offer a couple of options to people who contact you.

Then, create a notice that says:

Announcing the Formation of a New
Fibromyalgia Support Group
Please call xxx-xxxx or e-mail xx@xxx.com
Call between 11 a.m. and 2 p.m.

Be specific about the time you wish to be contacted. If your brain only functions between 11 a.m. and 2 p.m. (like mine), say so. If people are interested, they will find a way to call you at that time. Have a couple of times and a location available and ask what works best for the caller. Get a name and a phone number so you can call back to confirm a date and time after speaking with a few interested people.

As with any new venture, if you want to attract people, you must advertise. Send a notice to each rheumatologist's office in your area and to as many GP offices as you can cover. Call them first to tell them what you're doing. The office staff will then be more likely to post your notice when they discover it in the mail. Also, ask for ideas for other people to contact or other places to hang your notice.

Grocery stores, libraries, health clubs, and health food stores are all places that are patronized by persons with fibromyalgia – in other words, everywhere! If your homeowner's group has a newsletter, post it there. Contact every other neighborhood organization in your area. Most of them have newsletters. If the company you work for has a newsletter, post it there.

Be sure to tell your friends and neighbors about your group formation. They may also have access to newsletters where they work or they may know someone who knows someone who may be interested. Also, ask each interested person who contacts you to make additional notices and post them in other places you may not have covered.

THE ORGANIZATIONAL MEETING

First Order of Business: <u>Ask for a co-leader (or 2)</u> It's much less stressful to lead a group if you know someone else is sitting in the front seat with you. Also, if you're not feeling well, it's not such a disaster if you need to miss a meeting.

DECISIONS TO MAKE

<u>Who to Include:</u>

Decide whether your group will include people with similar illnesses like Chronic Fatigue Syndrome (CFS), lupus, etc. These illnesses are very similar and often overlapping. People who suffer with one can often benefit from the experiences of people who suffer with another.

<u>Membership/Call List</u>

Get names, addresses, e-mail addresses and phone numbers of all attendees, as well as the best time of day to call each one. Set up an e-mail list as well as a phone tree so that each member gets reminded two times before each meeting. Then, as the leader, you just need to contact the first person on the list who calls the second person on the list, etc. If no copy machine is available, take the member list home and get copies made before the next regular meeting. A one or two dollar per meeting fee is helpful to pay for future paper and copying costs.

<u>Assign Functions</u>

It is important to have as many members as possible feel they are necessary to the functioning of the group. Being assigned an ongoing task is one of the best ways to accomplish this. Here are some useful assignments to consider.

- <u>Researcher</u> - This task is not as difficult as it sounds. Lots of people spend time on the Internet every day. It's no hardship for them to subscribe to a site that lists new information about fibromyalgia or to read a blog written by someone who does.
- <u>"Doctor Book" Keeper</u> - Assign someone to keep the "doctor book". These are just comments made by members for the benefit of other members who are considering a change of doctors. It should consist of facts rather than opinions. Pertinent entries might include "Doesn't prescribe narcotics" or often keeps you waiting more than an hour" or "Good listener".
- <u>Roster Keeper</u> - Maintaining a current and accurate list of members is vital to the success of the group. This is the way information is disseminated – about meetings, about members in need, anything and everything of importance to the group. There should be a phone number and an e-mail address for each member. A reminder should be made at the beginning of each meeting to report any changes to the Roster Keeper.
- <u>Program Scheduler</u> - After the group determines what topics they would like addressed, this list could be delegated to the program scheduler who would then begin contacting possible

speakers on the various topics. Sometimes this task is assigned to the group leader.

- Refreshment Coordinator - There's lots of room for variation here. Some groups elect to forego refreshments completely – too much trouble. Some groups are limited because of lack of facilities – no coffeepot or running water. The least desirable arrangement is for anyone to bring something whenever they want to. This results are that some meetings will have no refreshments and some meetings will have food that goes to waste.

- Publicity - The success of your group is directly related to the number of people who know about your meetings. Ensuring that a meeting announcement is printed in the paper each month, announcing the guest speaker and his topic, and inviting the public to attend is very important. The local newspaper and radio stations need to be called to see if they transmit community notices and what the cutoff date is. Included in the announcement should be the statement that "Meetings are fragrance free".

- Absentee Follow-up - Because of the nature of fibromyalgia, even the most interested group members will miss meetings from time to time. Assigning a member to call the people who missed a meeting is an important function. In the best case, the absentee either had other plans or was feeling ill, is feeling better, and knows that she was missed. In the worst case, the absentee is feeling really poorly and could use assistance in the form of grocery shopping, transportation, or a phone call to cheer her up. In either case, the caller can e-mail the rest of the group to find her the help she needs. This is important: Members should always have the option of not being called when they miss a meeting. Some people prefer to be left alone when they're feeling bad, and they have plenty of family members to fulfill their needs if necessary. Even a caring phone call may feel like an intrusion.

DETERMINE MEETING FORMAT

Guest speakers or discussions? The group must decide if they wish to have guest speakers or limit meetings to group discussions only. My experience has been that some of each is best. Having a guest speaker at every second or third meeting is a good plan, but this choice should be put to a vote.

It's also best to make decisions about group discussions in advance. A specific topic for discussion makes a meeting run more smoothly. The individual chapters of this book, for instance, are an excellent source of meeting topics and one reason I decided to write a second edition of Tender Points. Decide at the previous meeting what chapter will be discussed at the next meeting. People can then be prepared with a story to share rather than having to think of something spontaneously. Each member should be limited to a specific amount of time (Five minutes works well.) to comment on that topic. An egg timer is useful for this purpose. Keeping on one topic and limiting the discussion time for each member usually results in a more positive outcome than trying to address many different issues at each meeting.

CONDUCTING A MEETING

It's not as difficult as you might think, especially if you have a co-leader. The leader should call the meeting to order, welcome the attendees, and thank them for coming. After delivering any items of interest to the group, the meeting guidelines should be read for the sake of new attendees and to remind ongoing members. Then let each person give their first name and mention one or two of her most pressing problems if she would like to. Be sure to mention that this is optional. Also be sure to mention that according to the group guidelines, no one except the invited speaker talks for more than 5 minutes at a time.

The leader should summarize the issue to be discussed. One idea would be to read a chapter of this book, ask the first discussion question, then start the discussion. One group member after another can offer input – but only for 5 minutes each. The leader should announce when the 5-min. limit has been reached and urge members who wish to hear more to contact the speaker after the meeting or by phone or e-mail. Then move to the next person. Explain that although you don't mean to be rude, limiting response times is essential to dismissing the meeting at the time announced. This may be very necessary for many people who have issues like transportation, babysitting, etc.

MEETING GUIDELINES

Here are some rules that can help make your group more successful:

<u>Keep the Tone Positive and Upbeat.</u>

Yes, people need to vent, but that's best done among friends, one-on-one. Listening to a lengthy tale of woe is not usually helpful to the group at large.

<u>No Doctor bashing during meetings.</u>

Such discussions tend to take over the agenda and lend an air of negativity to the group – exactly what you want to avoid. It is far better to set aside 10 minutes after the end of each meeting for a "doctor discussion" if the members want one. This is the opportunity for members to find a new doctor or just to complain about the one they have. It is beneficial for someone to monitor this group and keep a "doctor book" containing both good and bad (but only factual) comments about each local doctor.

<u>Meetings are Fragrance Free.</u>

Many fibromyalgia sufferers are extremely affected by odors – even very nice ones (Multiple Chemical Sensitivity). Hairsprays, deodorants, perfumes, shampoos, conditioners, etc., - anything with a strong scent can be very irritating to many group members.

<u>Time limits are strictly enforced.</u>

People with pain problems have difficulty sitting through lengthy meetings. No meeting should last longer than 90 minutes. If you don't adhere to your schedule, attendees will be looking at the clock and will be reluctant to return. It's always a good idea to leave the group wanting more – rather than being happy to leave.

All discussions are confidential.

Every member should understand that anything said in a support group meeting stays in the support group meeting. With that rule in place, people will feel more comfortable expressing their feelings without the worry that their problems will be heard all over town.

5-Minute maximum on any member discussion.

Interested parties can continue any discussion that passes the time limit either after the meeting, by phone or by e-mail. It's the leader's job to say, "It's time to move on to the next member, but anyone who has additional feedback for Jane or Mary may e-mail them at xxx@xxx.com. This is another good reason to keep the membership list current and accurate.

Name Tags are required.

Nametags are vital for people who commonly struggle with fibrofog. They are especially important when the group is new or whenever a new member is in attendance. We all like to know the name of the person we're addressing, and many of us have memory issues. Inexpensive sticky labels are available at office supply stores. Ask each member to fill one out when signing in.

PROGRAMMING

- This is the area that can make or break your group. If you can provide the kind of information your group wants to hear, you will keep your members coming. If you don't, you won't. It's that simple.

- The role of the group leader should be to learn what kinds of information the members are interested in, and to provide that kind of information. Doing this will attract new members and keep the current ones coming back month after month.

- Members should be polled to find the topics of most interest to the group. To do this, make a list of every topic you can think of and distribute this list to the members. Instruct them to circle the ones they like, and be sure to leave room for write-in suggestions as well. Do this at the initial organizational meeting and do it again annually for the benefit of any new members or for people who have new ideas.

- Here's an example of the type of list you may wish to use.

ADA (Americans with Disability Act)
Acupressure
Acupuncture
Anxiety
Aromatherapy
Assistance animals
Breathing Techniques
Cannabis
Chiropractic
Depression
Ergonomics
Homeopathy
Massage Therapy
Meditation
Nutrition

Pain Management
Reflexology
Social Security Disability
TMJ & Dental problems
Tai Chi
Qi Gong
Yoga therapy
Other:

_____

_____

_____

_____

_____

_____

_____

_____

After the lists have been collected and compiled, the leader or the program scheduler can begin the search for knowledgeable speakers on the various topics selected. It is important that speakers understand the time restrictions for your group. Be sure to explain that you will be watching the clock and will point to your watch when their presentation must be concluded.

Other support groups in your area may be a good source for programming. Even if their focus is an unrelated illness, they may have many of the same interests as your group does. For example, a yoga therapist may be an appropriate speaker for a fibromyalgia group as well as a group for people with back problems.

If there are no support groups in your area and you don't have the inclination to form one yourself, or if you just don't have the strength to get dressed and get yourself to a meeting on a regular (or even irregular) basis, consider joining an on-line chat room. One that has been in existence for many years is called fibrohugs.com. They charge a fee of $5 per month or $36 per year. Patients Like Me.com has a well-used chat room for fibromyalgia. Daily Strength.com also has an online support group for FM as well as nearly any illness you can imagine.

For those of you who don't have access to a support group, for those of you who are frustrated by the enormous amount of information on the internet and elsewhere, and especially for those of you who don't have a fellow sufferer to talk to, I want you to know that people with FM can and do get better.

More importantly, I want you to know you're not alone. This book is my attempt to share with you what I have learned through my long acquaintanceship with FM. Let me be your "fibro friend" and I will tell you what I know.

Discussion Questions:

> *How did you find your support group?*
> *What would you change about this group?*

Chapter 26

Congratulations, You're SSA Disabled

If there's anything more demeaning than not being able to do your job for health reasons, it's trying to convince the Social Security Administration (SSA) that you can't. Even when you explain that you spent several years attending college at night while working full time and raising a family in order to get this job, they still don't believe you. Even when you document the promotions you've had and the commendations you've earned for exemplary performance, they still don't believe you. Instead, they assume that every applicant is a slacker, and they do all they can to make you believe that you are one, too.

Although many years have elapsed since I went through this process, support group members who have done it recently tell me that not much has changed. So, allow me to share my experience with you.

The application process, designed to be time-consuming and degrading, begins when you call to make an inquiry. At that point you're given a telephone appointment in several weeks time. Prepared to finally tell your story, you assemble all your medical information and answer the phone at the designated time. This conversation turns out to be with a clerk who has the IQ of a cabbage and knows absolutely nothing about medical issues. His sole function is to verify your name, address, social security number, and the fact that you haven't worked in 6 months. Don't try to give him any more detail. The form he has won't accommodate that. He'll say you'll be receiving information in the mail within two weeks. So you wait.

The paperwork arrives, and you fill out the forms, listing how you spend your day, who you see, where you go, what symptoms you have, who your doctors are, and why you think you can't work. You mail them in, and then you wait.

Once the SSA receives your paperwork, different paperwork will be sent to each of the doctors you listed. As this paperwork is not high priority for any physician, a delay is almost inevitable. So, you wait some more. It takes several phone calls to each of your doctors and an excellent relationship with his/her office staff to urge them to fill out the forms.

Eventually a letter arrives from the SSA advising you of an appointment for an examination by their doctor at a time and place approximately two months in the future. You go. You get examined. You're encouraged by your conversation with their doctor who appears to understand fibromyalgia and empathizes with your condition. Then you wait some more.

Some months later, the SSA sends you a letter stating that they have determined that you are not disabled and that you are capable of working full time. "WHAAAT????? I haven't been out of bed for more than two hours a day for the last week except to visit my doctor. There must be some mistake!!!!!" It was no mistake.

This is just routine, the SSA's modus operandi. Receiving an official turndown is a real shock to someone who doesn't understand the system. Only later did I learn that every application is refused the first time. You could be in a coma, unable to move a muscle, with only hours left to live, and your initial application for disability would still be denied. It's just the first of many ploys used to lengthen the process and ultimately discourage people from receiving the benefits they deserve.

After this refusal, many people think that's the end of it. So they grit their teeth and go back to work, disabled as they may be. I knew a young man who worked every day in excruciating pain after returning from Vietnam with a hypodermic needle broken off in his spine. His condition was inoperable. When his application was rejected by Social Security, he thought, "I must not be as bad off as I thought I was. I guess I'm just a complainer." He went back to working in pain, struggled with prescription drug abuse and alcoholism and passed away three years later as a result.

Could there be something wrong with this system? There is. It's broken, badly, and riddled with abuse. There are probably more people collecting benefits fraudulently than there are legitimately. But, don't let that sad fact stop you from applying if you truly cannot work any more.

You can't even apply for SSA benefits until you've been unemployed for 6 months. With bills to pay and families to support, lots of suffering people can't afford to play the government's waiting game. I was one of the fortunate ones. I worked for a large corporation which assisted me with the process, even providing me with an attorney to facilitate the Social Security application. On the second try, I received my benefits. Sound too good to be true? It was. But I was too naive to know it at the time.

Many people are denied again on the second try. At

this point most give up and go away. This is a huge mistake. It's only on the third try that you're given an opportunity to speak with an Administrative Law Judge. Scary as this sounds, it's not a bad thing. Unlike the SSA clerks, the judge is an intelligent human being who will read your physicians' findings, ask pertinent questions, and observe your physical condition. With or without representation by an attorney, everyone I know who was truly ill and persevered to this stage was awarded their benefits by the judge they saw.

The thing about the application process many applicants fail to understand is that the SSA does not want to know how bad your health problems are. I said it before, but it bears repeating: The clerks who read your application forms have little or no understanding of medical issues. At the third stage of the process, all they want to know is how your health problems prevent you from working.

For example, it was only interesting that because of fibromyalgia and rheumatoid arthritis I suffered incredible pain in most of my body that could only be controlled with narcotics that made me too groggy to think or to work. This information wouldn't impress the SSA at all. The important thing for them to know was that my pain was aggravated by repetitive motion, repetitive motion was necessary for computer use, and computer use was required for every professional job in today's workplace.

This distinction is crucial in order for your application to be considered. You must focus on why you can't work. Nothing else. SSA clerks are not trained to evaluate medical conditions. So don't go into detail about how bad your symptoms are. No one will care but you. Just focus on how your symptoms make it impossible for you to work – not just the job you're doing, but any job.

Each of your doctors must make this distinction as well. Although you would hope that your doctors' input is reviewed by SSA's medical personnel, this information will first be read by the clerks on the Administrative Law Judge's staff, should you get to that stage of the process. Even though the connection between your symptoms and your inability to work seems perfectly apparent to you and to your doctor, that connection must be made in writing in words a 6th grader could understand. Without this, no matter how ill you are, it's almost certain your application will be denied.

Speaking of doctors, it is imperative that you have a report from a rheumatologist included with your application forms if your reason for filing is fibromyalgia. For whatever reason, the SSA believes that only a specialist (i.e., a rheumatologist) can diagnose FM.

If you feel that disability is the best choice for you, be sure to find a physician who is on your side. Be aware that there are physicians who don't believe in disability for their patients under any circumstances. Some are just unwilling to fight the battle. Others have the mistaken notion that once a person is declared disabled, he is apt to sit at home and do nothing with his life; therefore, his condition will deteriorate. My personal experience and that of other long term fibromyalgia patients I know says that this is absolutely untrue.

Once you've been relieved of the daily agony of working while in pain and/or exhaustion, you have the time and energy to devote to your own wellness. You can exercise at the time of day when your body is most rested. You have the time and energy to do yoga or to practice meditation. You can read and learn and practice helpful therapies. You can join a support group and gain information from others who've been where you are. In short, you can focus on living well rather than on making a living. And you will begin to feel like a human being again.

Yes, fighting the eligibility battle with the Social Security Administration is a horrible experience. But it's just another battle. People with FM fight battles every day - against pain and fatigue and fibrofog. This is a battle you can win - if you have perseverance and the cooperation of your general practitioner and your rheumatologist.

Discussion Questions:

> *What was your experience like when applying for disability?*
> *What questions do you have about the process that this group could help answer?*

Chapter 27

Private Disability Insurance (or Here come the FCE's)

When my fibromyalgia symptoms became so severe that I could no longer work, I took comfort in the fact that I had purchased a long-term disability policy through my employer when I began working there 14 years earlier. This meant that I would receive a monthly check for 60% of my salary until I reached age 65. That, in addition to my Social Security Disability payment would cover my expenses. I considered myself blessed.

After these payments were established, I set about to make my life as good as it could be. I found that life without work was very lonely. After having worked at the same company for all those years, my friends were all former co-workers. Yes, we still spoke on the phone and met for an occasional lunch. But, as time went by, we had less and less in common. I tried volunteering, but soon realized my good days were too few and far between to fulfill even those minimal obligations.

Caring for my large home in snowy upstate New York was a tremendous burden. My home was on 3 floors, bedrooms upstairs, laundry in the basement. The house was draining my limited energy, the gloomy weather was deepening my depression, and my identity was wrapped up in a career I no longer had. In a desperate attempt to improve my health, I sold my home of 25 years and moved clear across the country to California. A radical move like this is not for everyone. In fact, it nearly wasn't for me. My strength was zapped so severely that I spent most of my first month in sunny California in bed.

For me, however, the end result was worth it. This move was the very best thing I could have done for myself. I now live in a climate where I don't need to worry about slipping on the ice, shoveling my sidewalk, or hiring someone to plow my driveway. I get out to walk nearly every day. The increase in the number of sunny days is directly proportional to the decrease in my depression.

Six months after my move I was notified by Cigna Insurance that my disability benefits were being cancelled. Their reason was that because fibromyalgia was a psychological disorder my policy was limited to only two years of payments instead of until retirement. A psychological disorder??? Because depression was one of my symptoms, they used it as justification for their nonpayment.

Fortunately, times have changed. It is now well established that FM is indeed a physical condition, so this will not happen to you today. When I protested, I was introduced to the Functional Capacity Exam (FCE). Simply put, an FCE is a tool used by insurance companies to prove that you can work - even when you cannot. It is a two-day test administered by a Physical Therapist hired by the insurance company to determine whether you can perform simple tasks. It makes no mention of stamina, effort required, or after-effects of doing these tasks. It has absolutely no bearing on the kind of work you did. The results are the accepted standard used to determine whether or not you qualify for your insurance benefits, which according to the policy wording is "the ability to perform any job for which you are qualified by education or experience".

After a sleepless night, I awoke the morning of the test feeling weak and wobbly with two fingers on my right hand so swollen and painful that I was barely able to dress myself. I arrived at the testing site wearing my house slippers, requiring assistance to tie the athletic shoes they required I wear for the procedure.

I was completely unable to perform many of their tests such as picking up small plastic disks and placing them in a cup, carrying a heavy box from one end of the room to the other, and walking on a treadmill - because I couldn't hold on with my right hand. At one point, my knees buckled and I nearly fell down a flight of concrete steps, also part of the testing. I'd say I failed with flying colors. A copy of the test results I received in the mail confirmed that I had not passed and was, therefore, still considered unable to work.

Much to my surprise, a month later I received a second letter from my insurer that said, in effect, "The results of your FCE indicate that you are no longer disabled. Effective immediately we are terminating your benefits." Unfortunately for them, my copy of their FCE results said just the opposite, so they had no choice but to reinstate my benefits. Such audacity! They were so certain that the physical therapist they hired on their behalf would provide the results they wanted that they sent a notice of termination without even reading the test results!

Unfortunately, my reinstatement was only temporary. Six months later, a second FCE was scheduled, this time with a different physical therapy organization – also hired by the insurance company. The test was nearly identical. Nothing pertinent to the jobs I was "qualified to do by education or experience" (their wording in the policy) was tested.

Here's my advice. First, have someone drive you to the exam. Never drive yourself. If you do, it will be noted that "Subject is well enough to drive to and from the exam." It's just another strike against you. If you live alone and all your friends and family work, call Uber or a taxi.

Second, no matter how friendly the therapist appears, be aware that she is writing down everything you say, and that whatever you say can and will be used against you. If you mention that you occasionally have a good day or two, that will be noted. Her official report (a document she is being paid by the insurance company to create) will say, "Subject admits to being capable of working part time."

Third, create your worst rather than your best performance. Remember that you never know when your worst day will be or if every day may become your worst day. The insurance company is using every means at their disposal against you. You must do the same.

Here are a few suggestions: The day before the exam, do any and all physical activities that normally have negative effects on you. If grocery shopping normally does you in, do it the day before the test. If stair climbing is your problem, climb as many stairs as you can find. Engage in some repetitive activity and do it until you've reached the limit of your pain tolerance. Push all your capabilities as far or farther than their limit.

You probably won't sleep well the night before the exam due to worry or anticipation, but don't do anything to induce sleep. If at all possible, take no medication the morning of the test. You can take your meds when you get home. Remember your goal!

Keep in mind that the FCE is a 2-day exam. Doing poorly on the second day won't require any thought at all. You'll be completely zonked from the stress and activity required the previous day. Struggling to perform will not be a problem. It will be a given.

I can't emphasize enough that whatever you manage to do, whether it's a struggle for you or not, will be noted as your normal performance. They will assume that if you can do it one time, you can do it repeatedly for an 8-hour day. They have no way of knowing that it hurt you to do it even once, or that doing it took every ounce of strength you had, unless you tell them or don't do it. So be sure that you do tell them or don't do it. Being "unable" is perfectly acceptable – even though it is so contrary to how we live our lives, struggling to be like everyone else, trying as hard as we can and suffering for it later.

Also, ask to rest when you feel the slightest bit fatigued. Refuse to resume their activities until you feel completely capable. If you reach a point where you can't go on, don't be afraid to say so. They will just postpone the remainder of the testing for a day or two.

I have concluded that this test was originally designed for and assumes that every person they test is a potential assembly-line worker. There is no opportunity to explain that repetitive motion causes you pain and debilitating muscle spasms – or that profound fatigue sets in after an hour of physical effort and that the fatigue makes your vision blurred to the point where you cannot read. The same test is administered whether you were a former nuclear physicist or a goat herder.

As you can see, the entire FCE process is a sham that is horribly skewed in the insurance company's favor. You are at a terrible disadvantage. As awful as it feels, you must do your absolute worst if you're to have any chance at all. As in any battle, the only way to win is to know your enemy. Now you do.

Hand in hand with FCE's are the investigators hired by the insurance company. They follow you around and film you doing the chores of daily living and interpret them as being capable of working. Once they decide to stop paying your benefits insurance companies will stop at nothing to prove you don't deserve them.

Even engaging in doctor-recommended exercise can be used against you. I was followed into the YMCA where I minimally participated in the Arthritis Foundation's Twinges in the Hinges program in their warm water pool for about 20 minutes. I then took a leisurely shower and chatted with some fellow support group members in the locker room about therapies we'd tried for knee pain. The official report read, "She worked out at the Y for over an hour."

If the insurance company's surveillance films don't produce anything they can use against you, they will edit them so that they do. For instance, my insurance company used a video tape of my taking a walk, another activity prescribed by my rheumatologist. The camera registered the date and the time I left home and filmed me walking for about 5 minutes. The next frame showed the date and time I returned home, which was one hour later. What the film didn't show was the part in between when I sat in the sun on a park bench for 45 minutes and watched the kids play at the playground. That part was edited out, and the investigator's written report read, "Subject took a one-hour walk." Don't underestimate the lengths to which these people will go.

The insurance company said the second FCE results (which were nearly identical to the first, except that I didn't fall down the stairs) and their surveillance photos supported their conclusion that I was capable of working in a sedentary position for an 8-hour day. Once again my benefits were terminated. This time it was permanent.

I have since learned that my next move should have been to contact the Consumer Complaint office of the state department of insurance. All insurance companies must comply with strict oversight from them. In fact, some companies are required to provide office space for state insurance representatives. If I had known such an office even existed, I certainly would have called them. However, I was uninformed, and I did not. Had I done so, I'm certain their ruling would have been overturned and my benefits would have gone on until I reached age 65 as I expected them to do.

Instead I learned about ERISA, which stands for Employee Retirement Income Security Act. Talk about misnomers!! This act was originally established to set standards for voluntary pension and health plans for the protection of employees. It has since evolved into a tool the Insurance companies utilize by using the wording it contains to weasel out of paying claims they rightfully owe.

Under ERISA, I had the right to appeal the insurance Company's decision, so I did. After nearly 9 months of intensive effort (mostly by me, not the expensive attorney I hired) an in-depth, medically-documented, 98-page appeal was produced. It included reports from all my past and present physicians, test results, lab results, occupational studies, x-rays, even input from several additional specialists who had examined me and concurred with the opinions of the rest of my medical team. All of this data supported the fact that I was "unable to perform the duties of any occupation for which I was qualified by education or experience." In other words, by their own definition, I was disabled. The appeal was denied.

My only recourse then (according to ERISA) was to sue. I hired a second attorney who had an excellent track record as a fibromyalgia litigator. (A litigator is a lawyer who tries a case in court.) He agreed to take the case for a whopping 40% of the settlement. Outrageous! But, what choice did I have? Without his help, I would have received absolutely nothing after having paid those hefty premiums for 14 years.

I am pleased to report that my case was finally settled. Almost 2 years after they abruptly cut off my benefits, Cigna insurance company offered to pay me approximately 60% of what they owed me in a lump sum (of which the attorney took 40%). My attorney's advice was to accept this settlement offer, given the fact that judgments in fibromyalgia court cases were uncertain at best. It seems that many judges, like many doctors, aren't sure fibromyalgia is a real illness, no matter how many scientific studies they see.

I guess I should be grateful. I might have gone to court, lost my case, and ended up with nothing. But any gratitude I might have felt is completely overshadowed by anger. I am angry that insurance companies are allowed to use the results of an evaluation conducted by a physical therapist that they select and that they pay as a completely legal tactic to get out of paying what they rightfully owe. How could a physical therapist I just met be a better judge of my capabilities than doctors who had treated me and my illness for years?

I am angry that the ERISA laws that were created to protect employees actually protect the insurance companies instead. I am angry that this nightmarish appeal process took 2 whole years out of my life. I am angry about the sleepless nights and debilitating flares I suffered from the stress of it all. I am angry that the entire appeal process negatively affected my quality of life, not to mention my bank account.

Many people in a similar situation choose to give up and go away. I was tempted many times myself. Making tactical decisions that affect your financial future is challenging at the best of times. Trying to do so in the midst of fibrofog, exhaustion and pain is truly a nightmare.

If there is a lesson to be learned here, it is that it's possible to "win" your fight for benefits with an insurance company, but you must be prepared to fight long and fight hard. You must also be willing to accept the fact that "winning" may not get you what you're owed. First and foremost, contact your State Insurance Department if you feel you're being unfairly treated.

Discussion Questions:

> *How long was it from the time you filed until the time you received your first disability payment?*
> *Did you use an attorney to help with your claim? If so, who was it?*
> *Would you recommend your disability insurance company to others?*

Chapter 28

Personally Speaking

No one is going to discuss the really personal aspects of living with FM with you except other FM sufferers who feel safe in revealing the most embarrassing details of their life. In the past, the best place for this to happen was at fibromyalgia conferences sponsored by the National Fibromyalgia Association (NFA). These conferences were attended by doctors, physical therapists, nutritionists, researchers, as well as patients and their spouses/ significant others from all over the country. I learned more about living with fibromyalgia from the people I met at those conferences than I learned from all the books I'd ever read on the subject. There were informative lectures from morning till night as well as opportunities to sample new products and to intermingle with new fibro friends.

Unfortunately, the NFA has disbanded due to the severe health issues of its director. Given the millions of people who suffer with this illness, I'm hopeful that the NFA will be resurrected in another incarnation, and these conferences will resume in the future.

It was while sipping a coffee in the hotel lobby after the first lecture of the day at a conference in Columbus, Ohio that I learned the true value of attending such an event. A group from West Virginia happened to be seated on the couch next to me, all of them laughing so hard that tears rolled down their faces. Just witnessing their hilarity was enough to make me laugh as well. When they'd recovered enough to speak, they included me in their conversation as naturally as if they'd known me forever. That was typical of the sisterhood that existed there. The topic this group had been discussing was "wetting your pants while at work." Would I make this up?

Yes, that had happened to me, if you must know. But I'd never shared that experience, not when it happened, not when I left work in a big hurry, not even weeks, months, even years later, not even to my closest friends, none of whom had FM. I was much too embarrassed to ever mention it.

There they all were, talking about their wet underwear as if it was the most normal (albeit hilarious) event in their lives. It only took a few minutes of chatting with these women before I began recanting my own tales of horror, which suddenly became hysterically funny rather than a source of secret shame I'd carried with me for so long.

These women were real people like me with the same irritable bladder and other FM problems that I had. Most of them held responsible jobs. This particular group included an attorney, two accountants, a bartender and a retail owner. Some were single, some were married. One was the mother of five children under ten years of age, God bless her. They were all intelligent women, informed about their illness, and as determined as I was to learn how to live with FM the very best way they could. I could relate to these women as I'd never related to anyone in my life - and I'd only just met them!

Feeling renewed after our break, we all trooped in to the next session. As I looked around the room, I recognized my old friend, fatigue, on the faces around me. Much of the audience looked the way I felt. It was only the second session of the day, and already exhaustion was setting in. As this session ended, tape recorders blossomed all over the room. FM people are nothing if not resourceful. Those who had enough strength to attend another lecture carried with them several tape recorders belonging to others who had slipped away for a nap. For newbies like me who had not thought to bring recorders of their own, those who had them were more than happy to take names and addresses and promised to mail copies of the tapes they made. Without exception, I received every tape I requested (at no charge, not even for postage).

Yes, there were professionally recorded tapes of all the sessions available for sale. But they were very pricey, and most of us had blown our budgets just to travel to the conference. We didn't need additional expenses.

After the third session of the day, I slipped away for a rest, then returned in time for the conference luncheon. Not finding my newfound friends in the enormous dining room, I seated myself at a large, round table for ten. All of the women there, like me, had come to the conference alone.

The subject under discussion was pain medication. I listened as they described side effects similar to the many I'd had. Indeed, they were the very same side effects my doctors said couldn't possibly have been caused by the drugs I was taking. Emboldened by the morning's conversation, I made a rather personal admission. I announced that in my humble opinion the best painkiller was sex. It was cheap, it was pleasurable, and it had no side effects.

Agreement was unanimous. All of the married women at the table reported frequent, orgasmic sex with pain relief as a very big bonus. Anticipating increased pain and fatigue from sitting all day at lectures; one woman had brought her spouse along to the conference for that very reason. That got a big laugh!

We all admitted that we were highly sexual people and that sex did indeed relieve our pain. Although we knew of no scientific research on the relationship between sex and fibromyalgia, we speculated that because our bodies were hypersensitive to pain, they must be hypersensitive to pleasure as well. Lucky for us, the endorphins produced during orgasm are the very same endorphins that kill pain.

The married women in the group all agreed that sex was the glue that held their marriages together. Although this may be true for marriage in general, it is particularly so for FM marriages. It's not easy for a man to live with a chronically ill wife, but there are definite advantages if her illness happens to be FM. This is a wife who is extremely grateful for every sexual encounter. What a great ego booster for a man - being able to give his wife pleasure and relieve her pain at the same time - not to mention satisfying his own sexual desire as well! One woman said her husband wanted to know how he could find another woman with FM if and when she died or left him!

Of course, there are downsides as well. Greg Piburn, the husband of an FM sufferer wrote a heart-rending book called Beyond Chaos describing how FM destroyed his marriage and nearly destroyed him as well. It's a good book to read when you begin to feel sorry for yourself and wonder why your husband doesn't care any more.

Motivated by memories of "safe" sex/pain relief, the unmarried ladies were all doggedly determined to find a permanent relationship. But it's not easy! The process of dating is a unique challenge when you're hurting and exhausted, one I don't necessarily recommend.

Unfortunately, there is also a dark side to sex with fibromyalgia. It is called vulvodynia or genital pain. Sex may kill pain, but vulvodynia kills desire. However, don't despair. Help may be available.

If your symptoms are caused by vaginal dryness, a water-based lubricant can help. If you have thinning of the vaginal walls due to a lack of estrogen, hormone replacement therapy is readily available, although it can be a daunting task to find the form and the dosage of HRT that your body can tolerate. Your choices include natural products like Remifemin as well as products made from horse urine like Premarin and Provera. Personally, I can't help thinking we were not meant to put that stuff in our bodies. But if it works for you, go for it!

Keep in mind that painful intercourse may also be caused by trigger point pain, yeast or a bacterial infection. So, be sure to check it out with your GP or gynecologist. Don't try to self-medicate if you're not absolutely certain of the cause. And, today, physical therapy is available for gynecological problems. Be sure to ask about this with your doctor.

Sex is none too inviting if your other FM symptoms are acting up. There's nothing remotely sexy about IBS, and depression can rob you of every feeling you ever had. Sexual desire is often the first to go.

Discussion Questions:

> *How have you handled the personal challenges of FM?*
> *What's your best advice?*
> *Any tips to save time and energy?*

Chapter 29

Twenty Minutes a Day

No, I'm not talking about sex. That topic is covered in Chapter 28! I'm talking here about housework.

You may be surprised to learn that you can keep your home clean and tidy with 20 minutes of effort each day – whether you live in a studio apartment or in a multi-bedroom house. And you can divide that 20 minutes into 2 10-minute sessions if you wish! It takes some discipline to force yourself to do it, but once you've gotten into the habit it becomes almost effortless, no matter how fatigued or pain-ridden you may be. For me, first thing in the morning is best - even before I get dressed. For you, another time of day may work better.

Here are three things that make this process doable:

1. Making a list, keeping the 2 most important elements in mind
2. Dividing large tasks into smaller pieces
3. Pacing

Pacing is essentially resting before you get tired. Can you imagine anything more difficult to do when you're looking at a dirty house and you finally have some energy for a change? The discipline required to do only what is doable for you is what makes this program possible.

Dividing large tasks into smaller pieces is another discipline that's difficult to master. If the whole house needs vacuuming and you have the vacuum cleaner in hand, it's a challenge not to complete the job all at once. But, don't! Keep your eye on the clock or set a timer and stop when your 10 or 20 minutes is over. Tomorrow is another day.

I recommend making yourself a list of chores that absolutely MUST get done each week - like vacuuming, dusting, cleaning the bathroom. Then do a couple of those nasty things each day.

Divide the really tiring chores like vacuuming in half and do it in 2 days instead of one. If you've ever felt overwhelmed by a dirty or messy house, try this technique. It really works! It's essential to schedule a rest period of at least 20 minutes after you've finished. Resting is just as important as keeping a clean house.

Remember to alternate your hands while you work, even when you're doing something as simple as dusting. You'll suffer less repetitive motion injury if you do. Whenever possible, work sitting down with your legs propped up. For instance, carry clean laundry to your couch or bed, turn on the TV or some, prop your feet up and fold away.

I sit down at the kitchen table to peel or slice veggies, and I keep a barstool in my kitchen if I need to be standing at the stove or at the sink for any length of time. Otherwise, pushing a stool out of the way is more trouble than it's worth. If it's absolutely essential to stand, I open a bottom drawer and rest one foot on it. It's easier on my back that way.

A wheeled cart can be a godsend. I use mine to carry groceries from the car to the kitchen, to carry the laundry to the washer, or for anything else that's just too heavy or bulky to lug around myself. The only problem I have is deciding whether to leave my cart in the car or in the house for when I need it next. Of course, it's always in the wrong place when I need it! Perhaps two carts are better than one.

Here are a few other tips for saving energy:

- Organize. Whenever possible, store all the things you need for a particular job in one place. For example, keep bathroom cleaning supplies in a carryall container with a handle (i.e. cleanser, bowl brush, paper towels, window cleaner). Keep everything you need to wash the dog in a plainly marked container (i.e. shampoo, hairdryer, old towels, grooming brush).
- If possible, purchase a second vacuum cleaner (estate sales are great places for these) and keep one on each floor of your house (if you have more than one). It saves considerable energy wasted from lugging the heavy machine from floor to floor.
- Raise your work surface so you're not bending over. If there's a lengthy task you need to do while standing at the kitchen table, put a couple of books under the table legs. Better yet, construct a table at a comfortable working height somewhere in the kitchen area and use it whenever possible.
- Bend at your hips or knees- not your back.
- Lift by straightening your knees.
- Carry heavy objects close to your body. It causes less strain on your muscles.
- Avoid overhead tasks whenever possible.

- Determine your best time of day and schedule physically demanding tasks at that time.
- Be flexible. If 20 minutes is just too much on a bad day, work for only 5 and save your chores for the next day or the day after that.

And last, but not least: Delegate. Unless you live alone, be sure to include other members of the household in the housekeeping duties. Allow them to assist in making the task list and in assigning each task to the person who is best able to do it. If children are involved, let them rotate their responsibilities if they wish, but don't let them off the hook. They'll be grateful to you later in life when they have their own homes to keep clean and will know just how to go about it. The discipline they develop by doing a nasty chore even though they don't wish to do it will serve them well in the future. Never, ever, do all the work yourself because you feel guilty or because you feel you SHOULD. It's their home, too!

Over the years, I've learned not to waste any more energy than I absolutely need to on unpleasant chores like housekeeping. This way, there might be enough strength left over to do something enjoyable later in the day - like reading a book or walking or anything else that makes me happy.

Last, but not least: Keep in mind that no one ever died from a dirty house

Discussion Questions:

> *What part of housekeeping is your greatest challenge?*
> *What one thing would make it easier for you?*
> *What techniques have helped you keep on top of things?*

Chapter 30

So You Think You Want a Pet

W hen I grew up we lived in a flat on the second floor. This was my parents' excuse for not owning a dog even though I wanted one desperately. So we had a parakeet instead. His name was Piper. He learned to talk because my mother was home, and she talked to him all day. He also learned to get out of his cage. This my mother did not teach him. She was terrified of birds.

A week after we got Piper, my father had to come home from work in the middle of the day because Piper was loose and was terrorizing my mother. This is a whole lot more excitement than parakeets normally generate. Most of the time they just sit on their perches and chirp until you put covers over their cages at night. They're nice company if you don't want a pet to cuddle.

During a particularly low point in my life, I desperately wanted a pet to cuddle. Both my FM and my rheumatoid arthritis were at their peak, and depression ruled the day. My therapist thought a pet might help. Too fatigued to walk a dog, I opted for a cat instead, even though I'd never owned one or even spent much time with one. I saw an ad in the newspaper for a "mellow lap cat". It sounded perfect to me, so I bought all the cat paraphernalia and went to meet him. He lived with a rescue lady who had 26 other cats as well. All the others were picking on this one, so he needed to go.

As soon as I sat down, this cat jumped up on my lap and purred while I petted him. I fell in love instantly and said I would take him. On the way home there were human-like wailing sounds emanating from the cat carrier I had never heard before or since. No one had prepared me for this. I hurried home, put the cat into the guest room, closed the door and allowed him to explore his new surroundings as the rescue lady had suggested.

When I opened the door an hour later, the cat was nowhere to be found. However, the floor, the walls, and my new pink bedspread were all splattered with blood. When he finally skulked out from under the bed, the poor thing was licking several bloody places on his body where he had pulled out hunks of his fur.

This was definitely not what I needed. This cat had more problems than I did! Quickly donning a pair of leather gloves, I put the poor hissing creature back in the carrier and hightailed it back to the rescue lady as fast as I could. So much for me and cats!

Don't misunderstand. There have been lovely cats in my life since then. They all belonged to other people, and I've enjoyed them all immensely. Don't let my experience with one deranged kitty discourage you, but keep in mind that owning any animal may not be exactly what you thought it would be. In other words, be prepared!

And so I turned to dogs. My first was a springer spaniel puppy called Jessie. Jessie was a present from my well-intentioned son who bought her for me shortly after my first husband died. Jessie was adorable, but she was a puppy. And puppies are a lot of work, especially at 5 a.m. when they want to go outside to play in the snow, and you don't. Unfortunately, I was so emotionally distraught at the time that I could barely care for myself, much less a puppy. So, Jessie went back to the breeder.

Years later, after moving to Ca., remarrying and buying a house, I finally got a dog. After my previous experience, I knew I didn't want a puppy but rather a young, small, affectionate breed that didn't shed. After months of research on the internet, I decided that a bichon frise was the dog for us. After several more months, I found one at a rescue center. He was even a purebred. We named him Max.

Max was playful and affectionate and smart as could be. He loved to be with people, and he didn't shed a hair. However, Max refused to be housebroken and suffered from severe separation anxiety. Leaving him in his kennel when we went out resulted in bloody paws. Leaving him in a room with the door closed resulted in scratched paint and chewed moldings. Leaving him barking and scratching caused me severe anxiety and stress. This I also did not need. After nearly 3 months of trying to train Max and blaming myself for his poor behavior, Max went back to the rescue group from where he'd come.

I felt like a failure as a dog owner, but I learned a valuable lesson from Max. I learned that I really did want a dog in my life. I just needed to find one that suited my personality. Eventually, I did. His name was Charlie, and he was everything Max was not. Of no particular breed, he was calm and quiet, patient and snuggly. He adapted to any situation, and he lived to go for walks.

Plagued by extreme guilt if I didn't, I took Charlie for a walk every day. I just couldn't ignore that wagging tail and hopeful look. I walked on days I never would have walked before - even when I was hurting, even when I was exhausted. And I always felt better as a result. FM experts agree that stretching and exercise are the very best treatments, but motivation is hard to come by when everything hurts. Owning a dog provides that motivation.

Charlie improved all my FM symptoms, but particularly my depression. A little dog can make you laugh no matter how awful you feel. Charlie followed me around the house all day, cocked his head when I spoke to him, and sat on my lap in the evening. And spending more time out of doors is a bonus for a person with a chronic illness. It's easy to become housebound and isolated when healthier people don't understand our reluctance to accept invitations or our canceling commitments at the last minute. Eventually they stop inviting us. Dogs are great socializers, and walking in your own neighborhood is an opportunity to interact with people.

Regardless of the size of dog you're considering, think about a therapy, service or companion dog. There are many organizations that raise and train dogs to do many helpful things. One such organization is Canine Companions for Independence sponsored by the Lions Club. Another is Assistance Dogs International. You don't need to be blind, paralyzed or in a wheelchair to qualify for one. If you need a little help because of a physical or psychological affliction, your request for a dog will probably be fulfilled.

I was fortunate to be well enough to train Charlie myself to be a licensed therapy dog, even though his only official function was to prevent my claustrophobia and panic attacks on airplanes. However, if you don't feel up to doing the training, it can be done for you. And the dog will be happier for it. They love to have a job to do; they live to please. Another bonus is that once they've earned their badges and their vests, they can go anywhere you can go, even to restaurants or on airplanes. It saves you the stress of finding someone to babysit if you need to be away for an entire day or to take a trip.

If a therapy dog is not for you but you're considering a small breed of dog, you might investigate a Mexican hairless variety called a Xolos (pronounced sholos). They've been used as unofficial therapy dogs for hundreds of years because of their extreme body heat and docile personalities. They can be trained to sit or lie on your sore places to share their healing warmth with you. It's a lot like having a four-legged hot water bottle.

The downside of pet ownership, as any dog owner will attest, is their short life span compared to humans. An indoor cat you raise from a kitten lives an average of 12-14 yrs. Outdoor cats not so long. The median life span for dogs is 10-13 yrs. (more for smaller dogs, less for larger ones). Domesticated birds have the widest average life span, ranging from 10 years for parakeets up to 50-60+ years for macaws. It's definitely a factor to consider. Be prepared to fall in love with your dog, and be prepared to lose him as well. It's as painful as the loss of any human in your life – maybe more so. They do, after all, spend more time with you than any human does.

Another factor to consider is expense. For cats and dogs, costs begin with spaying, vaccinations, regular check-ups, and can escalate from there. My advice is to purchase health insurance for your pet. A monthly premium is easier on the budget than a bill for major surgery. SPCA and Nationwide offer policies that have adequately met our needs at a fairly reasonable price.

Being responsible for another living being is a very healthy thing to do if you can, especially for those who live alone and/or for those who are no longer working. Finding a reason to get up in the morning or to get dressed and start the day can sometimes be difficult. Knowing there's a hungry little creature waiting just for you can be the perfect answer. Be it a dog or a cat, a bird or a goldfish, sharing your day with a pet is definitely therapeutic. It adds another dimension to your life.

Our Charlie passed away from colon cancer three years ago, and we still mourn his loss to this day. We've spent countless hours searching rescue sites online as well as local shelters for a comparable replacement, but have not yet been successful. But we'll keep trying. For us, the benefits of owning a dog far outweigh the pain of losing one.

It may take a little doing to find the perfect pet for you. But don't be discouraged. Your "Charlie" is out there somewhere, and he's definitely worth the effort it takes to find him.

Discussion Questions:

> *How has owning a pet affected your FM symptoms?*
> *What's the funniest experience you've had with your pet?*
> *Would you recommend pet ownership for all fibromites?*

Chapter 31

Travel at Your Own Speed

When you're not feeling strong and healthy, the best place to be is at home. However, for those of us who rarely or never feel well, that's not always an option. At various times we must travel, either for family reasons, business reasons or when we just can't bear another minute of staring at our own four walls.

For some (young, old, healthy or sick), the very idea of traveling is so daunting that they opt to stay at home. Because my family lives far away, my choices are to stay at home and miss them, or get on a plane and do my best to arrive as healthy as I can.

My goal (and that of anyone traveling with pain and fatigue) is to do it in a manner that causes the least fatigue. To do so I take advantage of any and every assistance offered. Here are some tips that can make your journey more pleasant, keeping in mind that your main objective is to save your strength.

Let's start at the beginning. Before you travel, you need some reservations unless you'll be travelling by car. In that case, be aware a AAA membership comes with all the maps and travel guides you could possibly need in addition to much-needed assistance should you experience a car problem.

The state of train travel in this country is a real shame. European countries have it all figured out very nicely, but we don't seem to learn from them. Instead, we keep coming up with extremely expensive and impractical plans that get vetoed by taxpayers in nearly every state.

Our most common form of transportation is the airplane. If you haven't travelled in a while, you'll be in for a shock. What was once an enjoyable pasttime has deteriorated into a nightmare. It features long lines for checking your luggage and even longer lines for security - all with no place to sit for the elderly or infirm. Over the years, I've had to figure out ways to deal with this less than pleasant experience in order to make it doable for me. Let's start from the beginning and I'll share with you what I know.

Airline Reservations

If you haven't done much travelling, just making reservations can be daunting. I usually begin by visiting my favorite online airline first. (The one I like best is the one that doesn't have assigned seats and doesn't charge to reschedule a trip.) If they don't happen to fly where I need to go, then I visit one of the discount sites like Travelocity or Priceline. Once I learn which airline has the least expensive or most convenient times for me, I contact that airline directly. The reason I prefer to deal with the airline itself is that if there's ever a problem, you can get help right from the source. There are also consolidators who purchase entire blocks of seats from the airlines and may have seats left to sell at times when the airline itself does not. Booking your flight at least 3 weeks in advance usually guarantees the lowest fare. I've been told that Tuesday is the best day to book a flight, although I couldn't tell you why that is.

I've also been told that when shopping for flights, you should use "incognito mode" on your computer (Control/shift/N works on some computers. Yours may be different). Without it, prices will go up as you move from one site to the next.

Be aware that the discount travel sites charge your credit card the instant your reservation is made - even if your trip isn't for another 6 months. If you book your flight with an airline directly, they often don't charge your card until they issue your ticket.

Another thing to consider are the cancellation fees. Most airlines charge substantial fees for changing your reservation. It can be as much as $250, sometimes more than the cost of the ticket itself. It pays to shop around and to ask. With the unpredictability of FM flares, being able to reschedule might be worth a more expensive fare.

One thing I learned recently is that if you cancel an airline reservation the same day you book it, there is no charge. Early one morning I carefully booked connecting flights to and from Eugene, Oregon from Los Angeles for both me and my husband for the purpose of attending a granddaughter's graduation. After much discussion about the price, later that afternoon we concluded that the money we would spend could be better used to further her education. Decision made, I called the airlines. All flights were cancelled with no charge. What a relief! Given that my state of health changes from minute to minute, knowing this will be somewhat of a comfort in the future.

If the reason for your trip is a family emergency (a family member has died or is dying), always call the airlines directly and tell them the reason for your trip. Most airlines (American is a recent exception) offer special "compassion" rates and can squeeze you in on flights that appear to be sold out if you look on your own.

You'll be asked to provide some proof of the situation, but it's usually a document that's not difficult to obtain.

If you're booking an airline with assigned seating, always request a seat in the front of the plane when you make your reservation. Navigating down the aisle of a moving airplane can be quite a challenge on wobbly legs. Explain that you have mobility issues and ask if there's anything unusual that you should know about this particular flight - like stairs to climb to get on the plane from the tarmac or a long layover in a connecting city. I've been surprised by things like this more times than I care to remember.

To avoid the inevitable fatigue caused by travel, request wheelchair assistance at both your departure and arrival cities when you book your flights. It's improbable that a chair will actually be at the curb waiting with your name on it - although I've been fortunate enough to have it happen upon occasion. If there is none waiting and no one to ask, go directly to the counter (even if it means cutting in front of a long line of healthy people) and tell them you reserved a wheelchair. DO NOT wait in line.

If you have qualms about being pushed around in a wheelchair, remember this: That chair will be the ONLY place to sit while waiting in long lines at baggage check-in, again at security, at baggage retrieval, and at agriculture inspection and customs (if you're travelling to or from a foreign country). Wouldn't you rather save your precious energy for the things you wish to do once you reach your destination?

Never feel guilty or embarrassed about utilizing this service. Charging people lots of money for the privilege of waiting in long lines with no place to sit down is a lousy thing to do. The airlines know this, so they are happy to provide this service to anyone who asks for it. Just be sure to do so in advance.

Although the service is free, the cost is factored into the price of every ticket you purchase. You'll be paying for it whether you use it or you don't. So, you might as well use it. I always tip the pusher a few dollars, more or less depending on how helpful they were.

Pre-Boarding

When your wheelchair drops you off at your gate, your wheelchair pusher will ask the gate agent for a pre-boarding pass. These are given to people who need extra time because of infirmity or to people who have small children in tow. It provides an opportunity to walk down the narrow, sloping jet way at your own pace without being jostled or holding up a long line of people behind you. It also gives you almost guaranteed access to overhead baggage space right above the seat you select.

Because the plane is often empty when you board, you'll be tempted to select a seat in the front row due to the additional leg room it has to offer. It's best to refuse the temptation of that extra leg room unless it's a very short flight (under an hour). The first row has no place to stash your belongings within reach, and there often are no tray tables. If snacks are served or you've brought some food of your own, you'll be trying to eat it on your lap. Given the cramped spacing of aircraft seats today, this is no easy feat without elbowing the person seated beside you.

An aisle seat in the second or third row is a much better choice. Your gear (I suggest a backpack.) can be stored under the seat in front of you, and the amount of walking you'll need to do is still limited. Being seated on the aisle means you don't have to climb over people if IBS or an irritable bladder should become an issue.

On boarding the plane, ask a cabin attendant

(formerly known as a stewardess) for a glass of water (but only if it's from a can or a bottle) for taking medication. Also ask for assistance in stowing your heavy coat, etc. in the overhead bin. In addition to arriving in a wheelchair, you have just made it known that you have health issues, and the attendant will be a little more vigilant to your needs (should you have any) during the flight.

The Essential Backpack

The backpack is a traveler's best friend. I wouldn't travel without one - in addition to a small purse buckled at my waist. My backpack is my one personal item allowed (which gets stowed under the seat in front of me

My preference are backpacks with wheels, just in case there should be an occasion when I need to carry it.

These are the items it should contain:

- ALL medication - even things like Motrin, Imodium or TUMS. You never know when you'll need them, and baggage does occasionally get lost or stolen. It's possible to get replacement prescriptions phoned into a local drug store at your destination, but that takes a lot of time and effort that could be better spent on other activities.
- Excess clothing and/or shoes - On a single flight, the temperature can fluctuate 20 degrees or more between take-off and landing. Keep in mind that you'll be asked to remove your shoes at the security area. Slip-ons are preferable to tie shoes for this reason. If you absolutely must

have your walking shoes with ties for a later portion of your trip that day, carry them in your backpack.

- Address/appointment book or cell phone with the phone numbers of everyone you might ever need to call - including doctors, veterinarians, pharmacies, family, neighbors, etc.
- Food - Meal service on airplanes has become a thing of the past. Bring whatever you'll need to stave off hunger pangs, keeping in mind that if you're leaving or returning to mainland USA, anything organic will be confiscated. You may not bring in or take out fresh produce of any kind - even a cut-up fruit salad. Sandwiches, hard cheese, dried fruit and nuts are always good choices. To be on the safe side, plan for flight delays of 2 hrs. on each end of your flight. The only food you'll be offered on board will be salted nuts or pretzels. These will contribute to the dehydration you normally feel from just being inside a pressurized cabin. Being dehydrated will increase your jet lag and make you feel generally lousy. I always refuse these snacks or save them for another day.
- Drink - On-board water systems can be contaminated with bacteria, the last thing your already compromised immune system needs. Be sure any water you consume is water you purchased before boarding or water that comes from a bottle or a can. I always ask for the entire bottle or the entire can so I can be sure of what I'm getting.
- Cell Phone - This invention has really transformed the travel experience. If you don't own one of your own, borrow one for your trip. As soon as you have reclaimed your luggage

you can call the person or taxi who is picking you up. When you and your wheelchair arrive at the curb, your ride will be there waiting.

- Hygiene Mask - The air inside an airplane is loaded with bacteria and viruses. Even if you're not seated near someone who is coughing and sneezing, wearing a hygiene mask is an excellent idea. Lots of Japanese travelers wear them - not only as a protection against the germs of others but also as a courtesy when they themselves are sick. They can be purchased inexpensively at hospital supply stores and many drugstores.

- Make-up - If you're anything like me, you've spent years locating just the right products for your sensitive skin. Trying to replace them in an unfamiliar location would waste an enormous amount of time and energy you just don't have. Don't risk having them leak or melt or disappear from your suitcase. Keep them safely in your backpack instead.

Suitcases are another matter. If you have a carry-on-sized suitcase, store it in the overhead bin and avoid the wait at the baggage carousel. Most airline attendants will be happy to help lift your bag if you need assistance, especially if you arrive at the plane in a wheelchair. Many fellow travelers will also a helping hand. However, I was once rudely told by a steward, "if you can't handle your own luggage, you'll need to check it in." I've never flown that airline again. In addition, I wrote a letter to the management describing my experience. Now, to be on the safe side, if I plan to take a carry-on bag I pack it as lightly as I can.

Dressing for travel

To accommodate temperature fluctuations, dressing in layers is the best idea. Start with a short-sleeved t-shirt with a long-sleeved blouse over it, a sweater and a lightweight jacket on top. Elastic waists are easier than struggling with buttons and zippers on moving airplanes.

Be sure to have pockets on two sides. On one side, carry your Driver's License and boarding pass. Always use the same pocket for them so you won't need to search for them. Currently, photo identification and boarding pass (which can be printed at home the day before your flight) are required twice before boarding: once when checking in your bags and once when going through security.

In your pocket on the opposite side, carry several single dollar bills. A few will be used to tip the wheelchair attendant and you may wish to buy a newspaper and some bottled water after you pass through security.

Never discard your ticket stubs or baggage claim slips until your trip is completed and you've had an opportunity to examine your luggage. First, make certain that the luggage belongs to you. Many bags look alike these days. Then check to be certain nothing is missing from the inside. Items do get lost and/or stolen during the random inspection process if they're checked. If there's a problem, you'll need the numbers on the ticket stub in order to converse with the airline's customer service department.

If you flatly refuse wheelchair assistance due to pride or embarrassment or any other issue, consider purchasing a walking seat, also called a seat cane. They're especially popular in Europe. It's a lightweight, adjustable cane that becomes a folding seat. They are available at various places online, one of which is Travel Smith. Even if you don't use it, it weighs practically nothing, and it's a great conversation starter. You'll be amazed at how many people will ask where you got it when they see you sitting down and their legs are aching from standing in line. They will also be interested in hearing about your illness and glad to tell you about theirs.

There is also a new suitcase on the market that has a folding seat attached. Because the idea is so new, they are still very expensive. However, when other manufacturers copy the idea (and I'm certain that they will), it will become an affordable and indispensable item to own. I'll be the first in line.

If your budget allows, consider taking along an extra pair of legs. It could be a niece, nephew, neighbor or grandchild. It can be a treat for them and a big help for you. He/she can be your legs if and when they're needed.

If you don't have friends or relatives available, consider a therapy dog. (See Chapter 15 "So You Think You Want a Pet.") These dogs can accompany you anywhere - including airplanes and restaurants. They can give you much-needed stability on your feet and provide protection in unfamiliar places for those of us who are particularly vulnerable due to muscle weakness or fatigue.

And now a word about hotels: The place you choose to stay will be predicated by your budget and the convenience of its location. However, here are a few general tips that will apply no matter where you choose to stay.

- Always ask to inspect the room before you agree to take it. Large chain hotels often use very strong chemicals for cleaning. If the windows don't open or the room was previously occupied by a smoker, it could be a real problem for a person with MCS.

- If a room is not acceptable for any reason, ask to see another room.
- If it's a large hotel, ask for a room close enough to the elevator to minimize the amount of walking you'll need to do but far enough away to shield you from the noise of the arrival bell.
- If it's a high-rise building, ask for a room on a lower floor. Although I've only done a modest amount of travel, I've experienced 2 fire drills while staying in hotels. The first thing they do is turn off the elevators and tell everyone to walk down the stairs to the outside. I was once on the 22nd floor when it happened. I won't make that mistake again.
- If it's a motel, ask how close to your room you can park. Carrying heavy things back and forth can be very tiring.
- If after one night you find that the room was noisy from an adjoining room, hallway noise, elevator, traffic, ice machine or whatever, ask for a different room. If you've endured one sleepless night, you certainly don't want to endure another.
- If the room was too hot or too cold, ask to have the thermostat checked or to move to another room.
- In any instance where you are changing rooms because of a problem with the hotel/motel's facilities, it should be their responsibility to move your belongings. All you should need to do is pack. They should do the moving. If they refuse, not only should you complain to the general manager, you should write a letter to the CEO of the corporate chain if it's a chain operation.

Don't let your chronic illness keep you at home. If you enjoy traveling, you should go. If you're missing your loved ones far away, you should go. If there are places you've dreamed of seeing, you should go. Even if you're having a flare on departure day (a common occurrence after days of packing and preparation), you will likely feel better in a day or two. If you're travelling for pleasure, allow the first day at your destination to be a day of rest. Utilize the information listed here and remember to Travel at Your Own Speed.

Discussion Questions:

> *What was your last travel experience like?*
> *Have any tips to make travel a bit better for others in the room?*
> *What travel mistakes have you made that you won't repeat?*

Chapter 32

Those Nasty "Shoulds"

If you suffer from major fatigue as I do, you know that the key to survival is learning to pace your activities, to prevent exhaustion and to minimize stress. The fact is that our bodies have changed, our capabilities have changed, and we need to alter our expectations accordingly. However, too often we try to live by yesterday's goals which are unrealistic for our lives today. We often strive to achieve other peoples' expectations of our abilities. We do things because we feel we SHOULD. That's a really dangerous word for people with FM. It's just another word for guilt.

Here's an example of how the SHOULDS have gotten me into trouble.

Not long after having had surgery, I received the usual notices from the Red Cross Blood Bank saying that it was my responsibility to replace the 2 units of blood I received during the procedure. These notices arrived once a month for nearly a year along with occasional phone calls when the bank was getting low on my rare O-negative type blood. Finally, I decided I SHOULD do the honorable thing and fulfill my obligation.

On the next donation day at work, I was the first one there. Because I had never donated blood before, there was no way to anticipate the after-effects. I needed to be driven home where I remained in bed for the next 3 days, too weak to get up and walk around, too dizzy even to stand for long, too embarrassed to tell the people at work why I was home. Instead, I said I had the flu.

When I joined an FM support group many years later, I learned that my experience was quite common. Indeed, every fibromite there who had donated blood had a similar fate. My advice? Don't do it! Accept the fact that having FM makes you a poor candidate for blood donation - no matter how rare your blood type may be. I suppose I would make an exception in cases of extreme emergency; but, otherwise, I would opt to be the volunteer who distributes the orange juice instead.

When your child comes home and announces he's volunteered your cupcakes for the school party tomorrow, do you feel you SHOULD get out the baking tins

and the mixing bowl? If you're tired or in pain, don't do it. Supermarkets are open in the morning. Little kids don't know the difference. So what if the other mothers aren't impressed!

Your family is holding its annual reunion and you've been asked to bring the baked beans only you know how to make and everybody loves. Don't do it because you think you SHOULD. If you get great joy from baking beans and you have the energy, then do it. Otherwise, take Grandma Brown's to the picnic. Your family will forgive you. The more common problem is forgiving yourself.

This involves identifying what you're really feeling – which is guilt or a feeling of having done something wrong. According to quotes I've read from several learned psychologists, FM people tend to be hard-working, conscientious and compassionate. They typically experience excessive guilt because of how their physical symptoms and limitations impact their family and friends.

We need to realize that there are two types of guilt: reasonable and unreasonable. Reasonable guilt is when you have actually done something that had a negative impact on another. If this is the case, do what you can to amend the situation. Unreasonable guilt is when you haven't done anything wrong or selfish. It just feels like you have. This is the kind of guilt that can lead to psychological problems.

The first step to dealing with the guilt of FM (also known as the SHOULDS) is learning to identify it. As simple as this sounds, it's often difficult to do. It helps to ask yourself, "Why am I doing this activity that's zapping all my energy?" Once you've recognized an unhealthy behavior, you can begin to change it.

Something to consider is that we often project our own feelings onto others. We think, "I can't do the things I used to do. I don't like that. You must resent me for having to do more than me. Therefore, I'm a bad person and I should feel guilty." The cure for this, of course, is to ask the other person involved. You'll be surprised to learn that other people usually have more compassion for us than we have for ourselves.

One thing I know for certain is if you don't address the issue of guilt, it will fester and become bigger and more debilitating, eventually leading you to a lonely and isolated life. Discussing your feelings takes the problem out of the darkness and into the light where it can heal. In a 2007 article in Fibromyalgia Network News, Don Uslan, an experienced therapist in the Seattle area, recommends beginning the healing process by discussing one small issue with a trusted friend. Tell this person you're not looking for answers, you just need someone to listen. Then move on to another person and reveal another small problem.

Eventually you'll be able to discuss the really big issues with the most important people in your life, like your spouse or significant other. During these discussions, try to avoid self-blame. Rather talk about the things you <u>are</u> able to do. That will become a topic for consideration and the problem will become one you can work on together.

Learning to say no when you used to say yes can be a very big adjustment. One way to feel better about yourself is to make it a practice of sincerely and frequently thanking those who are picking up the slack created by your FM symptoms. Let them know that you're aware of what they're doing for you and that you're grateful for their extra efforts. It will also help them to feel good about themselves.

Public opinion and peer pressure can be powerful motivators. They can also be the source of unhealthy levels of fatigue. If you can learn to be more motivated by your body and your feelings and less motivated by what others might think, an enormous weight will be lifted from your shoulders.

We were all taught as children not to be selfish. But now we're adults, and we have fibromyalgia, a condition that limits our energy. Things have changed! It's perfectly ok to be selfish now. In fact, it's essential to our well being. The sooner you get the SHOULDS out of your life, the better you will feel.

Discussion Questions

> *What are some things you do only because you think you should?*
> *What are some alternatives you could use in your self talk instead?*
> *How have you learned to say "no"?*

Chapter 33

Fibro Primping

When it comes to appearances, fibromyalgia is a deadly disease. When you're in pain or when you're exhausted, the last thing you care about is how you look. However, it is also true (at least for me) that if you look better you feel better. Knowing that this is true for me, I've made some changes that have simplified my life and reduced the amount of time and effort necessary to make myself look presentable. Little things can make a big difference!

Because my neck and shoulders are particularly susceptible to pain, I'm very careful about the type of purses I use. I only buy the backpack type in order to distribute the weight evenly to both shoulders. The backpacks I use have wide shoulder straps, making them more comfortable to carry. I only carry in my backpack items that I'm certain I will need that day - in order to limit the weight. If it's not absolutely essential, my purse/backpack stays at home and I carry a credit card, driver's license, and car key in my pocket instead. For this reason, I now only buy clothes with pockets.

Speaking of neck and shoulder pain, if you're not sleeping on a down pillow, you're in for a wonderful surprise. Having had an allergy to feathers as a child, I stayed away from down pillows for years. Fortunately for me, I outgrew the allergy and happened to use a down pillow at a friend's house. I couldn't believe the difference in the pain level in my neck the next day. I've used a down pillow ever since. There's no scientific study to prove it works, but it's certainly worth a try.

Fussing with hair can be a nightmare when you have neck and shoulder pain. Holding up a hair dryer can be absolute agony. For this reason, I have a very short, very straight hairdo, which requires only a daily shampoo and a quick blow dry. On bad days, I even forego the dryer.

When I tire of looking at my short, straight hair in the mirror, I shampoo in some color so it looks a little different. The color also gives it some body. If the roots grow out before I have the energy to color it again, I just get a shorter haircut, and then most of it is gone. What's left looks like intentionally frosted hair until I get another cut or slap some more color on it.

Because I know that deciding on the right clothes to wear is a major chore in the morning, I try to keep my closet organized at all times. Short sleeve tops are hung on one side, long sleeves on the other. Same or similar colors are hung next to each other. Complete outfits are hung all on one wooden hanger so I don't need to search for each piece when I want to wear it. Items that haven't been worn in several months are relegated to a closet in the spare room, freeing up space so the remainder of my clothes are less crowded and easier to find.

Since my fibro symptoms began, I have consciously or unconsciously opted for comfort over fashion. Whenever possible, I choose clothing with elastic waistbands to allow for IBS bloat. My shoes have flat-heeled, thickly-padded soles which make walking easier on my knees and hips. I'll be the first one in line when they make sneakers to go with dresses. Until then, I'll wear mostly pants. They look less weird with my comfortable shoes.

While strolling through Macy's one day, I was approached by a cosmetics saleslady who offered to do a makeover on me. I must have looked particularly bad that day! This lady represented an all-natural, hypoallergenic product line so I agreed to let her do it. The outside of my body is as sensitive as the inside, so I have to be very careful about what I put on my skin. The prospect of sitting down in a comfortable chair while she painted my face was equally enticing.

What a shock it was to learn that I'd been using the wrong shade of lipstick and the wrong blush color all my life! When I saw the difference the correct colors made on my skin I was amazed. I immediately purchased a lipstick and a blush. Along with a little mascara, that's all I need to look presentable.

If you've never had a makeover by a professional, consider getting one done the next time you have enough energy to walk through a department store. It doesn't cost anything. The cosmetician would like to sell you her products, but you're under no obligation to buy them. If nothing else, there's usually a comfortable seat to sit on, and who knows? It might give you a lift as well.

In addition to looking good, fibromyalgia presents a challenge for smelling good as well. Soap and water should easily prevent body odor. The only challenge here might be the scents or the harsh chemicals that some of today's soaps contain. Be aware that anti-bacterial soaps have just the opposite effect. Because they kill of both the good and the bad bacteria, using those potent formulas can have a negative rather than a positive effect. Although I'm not a fan of deodorants, I know many people do need them and use them regularly. Because of the chemicals they contain, I'd tend to try other things first, such as baking soda which is an excellent odor absorber.

Mouth odor can be even more offensive than body odor – and it happens to be more common in people with fibromyalgia. The reason is that most of us have dry mouth - either from our illness or from one or more medications we're taking. Dry mouth is a major cause of bad breath.

To me, a true test of friendship is being able to tell a person that her breath smells. Actually there are subtle ways of accomplishing this. My usual technique is to offer the offender a breath mint. That usually prompts a question of, "Oh, my gosh, do I need one?" To which, I reply innocently, Possibly?..." Not everyone is fortunate enough to have such a person in their life. If you don't, you must be extra diligent about not offending people when you're near them. To test your own breath lick the inside of your wrist, wait a couple of seconds, and then sniff. It really does work!

The Fibromyalgia Dental Handbook, written by Dr. Flora Stay, DDS, offers several suggestions for fighting bad breath. One is to thoroughly clean the back of the tongue each time you brush your teeth. She also recommends chewing gum sweetened with xylitol after meals if you're not home to brush, drinking lots of water, and avoiding mouthwashes that contain alcohol. Alcohol is a drying agent and can worsen the problem.

Proper nutrition is also important for a sweet-smelling mouth. According to Dr., Stay, Vitamin A contributes to healthy mucous membranes in the mouth, so be sure to eat plenty of orange colored foods like carrots, sweet potatoes, cantaloupe and squash. Vitamin C will help prevent gum disease, so be sure to include plenty of citrus, green veggies and tomatoes in your diet as well.

A dry mouth sets us up for several dental problems in addition to bad breath. Gum disease, poor digestion, and increased decay can all result. Regular dental cleanings are even more important for us than for the general population. Consider scheduling your cleaning visits every 3 or 4 months instead of the usual 6.

The bottom line on looking good and smelling good is that it takes a little extra effort on the good days in order to balance out doing nothing on the bad days. When it comes to fashion, opt for feeling good instead of looking good. Fibromyalgia presents enough challenges without creating more just for the sake of appearance. Above all, be comfortable.

Discussion Questions

> *Have you altered your grooming habits after developing FM?*
> *What energy-saving tips can you share with the group?*
> *What products or ingredients in grooming products have caused issues for you?*

Chapter 34

I'm Still Me

While recovering from a hospitalization, I was issued a "Handicapped" placard for my car. Mostly, I used it when I was too exhausted to walk to the milk section in the back of the grocery store after a tiring day. Once someone left a note on my windshield that read, "You're not disabled. I saw you walk. Let someone else have that parking spot!" I actually felt guilty for weeks!

Only later did I rationalize the situation. What if I had a heart condition? I wouldn't have been limping from that either! Some people don't understand that not all disabilities are visible.

Because most fibromites look perfectly healthy, it is often a shock to people we know when proof of our disability emerges. The first time it happens can be traumatic for you as well. My first time occurred when I encountered a co-worker while I was riding an electric scooter in the enormous grocery store near my home one evening after work. Truth be told, the thought of just such a meeting had kept me away from these marvelous conveniences for a very long time. But, this particular day I had no choice. My legs were simply too weak to take me up and down the aisles, and I needed cream for my morning coffee.

Just as I feared, instead of the friendly greeting I would normally have received from this person, I was met with jaw-dropping dismay. This woman had sat opposite me at a conference table just hours earlier, but now she looked uncertain that she knew who I was. I was prepared to feel embarrassed, but I felt a whole lot worse than that. I felt ashamed. I felt socially unacceptable and totally misunderstood. I wanted to shout, "You have no idea how weak my legs are! I really need this contraption!!" Instead, I said nothing and behaved as though this mode of transportation was perfectly normal. Clearly uncomfortable, my so-called friend feigned an excuse to leave as quickly as possible.

I could usually put on a good face while at work. My fatigue didn't become limiting until early afternoon. That's when the fibrofog and the blurry vision set in. After that, every task was a struggle. If I were asked to do 3 things, without making a list, I was lucky to remember even one. I counted the hours until 5 o'clock when I could stop pretending. After 5, I became the real me - the me with fibromyalgia, the exhausted me who barely had enough strength to drive to the grocery store, much less walk up and down the aisles and stand in a line.

This encounter with my co-worker should have been a relief. Maybe, finally, the people I saw at work each day would begin to know who I really was, to understand the challenges I overcame just to show up each day. Instead, it made me feel bad about myself for the very first time.

The part that hurt the worst was that, up to this point, I had actually considered this fellow employee to be a friend. We worked for the same boss, occasionally lunched together, and attended many of the same social events.

Her disapproval was palpable, and I was devastated. Although we never mentioned the circumstances of that meeting again, our relationship disintegrated that day.

There were no more lunches. Conversations were strained and infrequent. The final straw came when I told her that I was leaving my job to go on disability. She tried to talk me out of it, suggesting that my condition was only temporary, that I should stick it out a little longer, and that I would soon regret having taken such a drastic step. There was no way for her to know how many years I'd been struggling or how desperate my situation had finally become. I was too good at covering it up.

That was the last time I ever saw her. She didn't answer my e-mails when I let her know I was moving out of town. A note with my new address received no response. Even though I long ago realized that this person hadn't really been much of a friend, I still feel the hurt.

You must be prepared for a wide range of reactions from both friends and strangers when you're using an assistive device such as a cane, a scooter or a wheelchair. Elderly people are always kind and anxious to offer assistance. They must realize how close they are to being in the same situation. Middle-aged people usually look away. Perhaps they're frightened to see what could lie ahead for them. Children are most often curious, wanting to know why you're sitting down or how fast your scooter can go.

For me, being on a scooter or in a wheelchair is a humbling experience. I am so grateful that these devices are available for my use but even more grateful that I can get up from the chair once I've left the Home Depot or arrived at my gate at the airport.

I've learned why there are organizations like "Wheelchair Pride." The world isn't made for people sitting down. So many things are missed at that level. Many people will be glad to completely ignore you. A lot of effort is required to get noticed and be heard.

Don't be frightened if a time comes when you can't function without a little assistance. I've had several times like that in my life, times when I needed a scooter to shop or to go long distances. For a while I carried a folding cane with a seat (available on the web for about $25). I took it with me wherever I went so that I could sit down when I needed to. I used it in lines at the bank, at movie theaters, department stores, etc. For almost a year, my legs wobbled so badly that I sat more often than I stood!

Fortunately, these were temporary symptoms. Difficult though it was, I continued to exercise, eat healthy foods, rest whenever possible and maintain my relationships with other people. In time, my strength returned, my pain ebbed, and I was able to physically and literally get back on my feet.

So, take my advice and use whatever resources you need to live your life the best way that you can. And try not to be intimidated by other peoples' reactions. If you should lose a friend in the process, that person wasn't much of a friend anyway. Continue doing all the healthy things you know you should do. Remember, this too shall pass.

Fibromyalgia is not totally disabling. You will not continue to get worse and worse forever. Rather, FM is a condition of remission. There will be good times and bad times. And you will be one of the few fortunate people on this earth who will really appreciate the good times when you have them.

One downside is that you'll become less tolerant of people who grouse about their ills all the time. You'll tire of hearing tales of their troubles, told to you in order to make you feel less bad about yourself. These folks mean well, but there's just so much tragedy one person can take!

Eventually you will seek the company of positive people, the achievers and the kind of heart. These are the people worth knowing. With enough knowledge about yourself and about fibromyalgia, you'll be one of them, too.

Discussion Questions:

>*Do you use any assistive devices?*
>*What reactions have you had from people you know?*
>*How did they compare to reactions from strangers?*

251

Chapter 35

And Then There Was One
(Grief and FM)

My first husband died suddenly of a heart attack in 1993. It was a terrible shock. I was still recovering from the loss of my mother who had died two years earlier on the very same day. I was totally devastated and unable to sleep, so I called my rheumatologist a few days later. He prescribed an anti-depressant for my immediate problem and gently advised me to prepare myself for a decline in my FM symptoms which had been under control up until that time. He said it was a well-known fact that stress aggravates the symptoms of fibromyalgia, and there's no greater stress than the loss of a spouse.

I was totally numb for the first few weeks, relying on friends and family to make my decisions. As if in a dream, I forced myself to exercise; yet I slept no more than 2 hours a night. I continued my habit of frequently swimming at the YMCA because being in the pool was the most comfort I had. The feel of the warm water surrounding me was the closest thing to the hugs I missed so desperately. And because swimming was an activity I had always done alone, there were no painful memories there at the pool to remind me of my loss.

About a month later I returned to work in an attempt to resume my life. My employers couldn't have been nicer or more understanding. They urged me to take all the time I needed. But I feared I'd lose my job if I took advantage of the situation. I no longer had a safety net. Because of my husband's lifelong battle with hypertension, there was no life insurance policy for me. My only source of support was my own job. I was truly on my own.

Episodes of uncontrollable crying erupted quite often and lasted for hours at a time. My brain was in agony, but my body was numb. As the months wore on, I awaited the increase in pain I'd been told to expect. It never happened. Instead, for the next year, I had a total remission of my FM symptoms. The very only thing I felt was grief.

Perhaps it was shock or that my total concentration was on learning how to live as a single person for the first time in my life. For whatever reason, time passed and my physical health remained stable. This was contrary to everything in the literature about fibromyalgia - and just another example of how different every case is. There are no absolutes in fibromyalgia.

Having a job to go to each day was excellent therapy as was the widows' bereavement group I attended. The loss of a spouse is so uniquely traumatic that only others in a similar situation can truly understand your feelings. I developed some close friendships in that group and learned some valuable lessons as well.

The most important thing I learned about grief was that you must go through it in order to get over it. You can't go around it by distracting yourself with increased activity or substance abuse. That only prolongs the process. Without a doubt, you will grieve the loss of a loved one eventually. The only question is when.

The sooner you do your grief work (yes, it is work, believe me), the faster you can begin to heal. An excellent book on the topic called, Getting to The Other Side of Grief, was an enormous help to me. This book and my bereavement group helped me through the worst of my grieving.

Although I'd never been a particularly religious person, I also found great comfort in my religious beliefs at that time. During one of my darkest hours, I visited my parish priest. I told him I felt completely empty, like there was a huge hole in my heart. He counseled me to "reach out." By doing so, he said, other people and events would gradually fill that hole. He was correct.

The loss of a loved one is only one of many losses suffered by most of us throughout our lives. Acknowledging that you have a life-changing illness like fibromyalgia is another loss. At some point you will grieve for the health you once had and the life you once knew. You will grieve for the things you enjoyed when you have to admit you'll never experience them again. And you'll grieve for dreams destined to remain dreams forever.

Unfortunately, grieving doesn't happen all at once. It's a process that can take weeks, months or years. Acknowledging your feelings is as important as is giving yourself permission to feel them. Sometimes it becomes necessary to intentionally invite them in, painful as this process may be. A therapist can be a wonderful help with this.

There's a very comforting and freeing document available at www.centerforloss.com written by Alan Wolfelt, Ph.D. Below is a brief version:

The Mourner's Bill of Rights

- You have the right to experience your own unique grief. Don't allow others to tell you what you should be feeling.
- You have the right to talk about your grief – or NOT.
- You have the right to feel any emotions. None of them are wrong.
- You have the right to respect your physical and emotional limits. Get plenty of rest. Listen to your body.
- You have the right to experience surprise grief attacks. Although frightening, they are normal and natural. Find someone to talk to about them.
- You have the right to use ritual. Funerals, wakes, candles, etc. Don't be influenced by others. Do what feels appropriate for you.
- You have the right to embrace your spirituality. If faith is important to you, use it. Be around people who share your beliefs, someone not critical of them.
- You have the right to search for meaning. You're entitled to ask tough questions like "Why me?" You don't need to accept stock responses like "It was meant to be."
- You have the right to treasure your memories. Don't ignore them. Embrace them – especially with others.
- You have the right to move forward and heal. It will take time. Be patient with yourself.

Recovery will be painful. But, in time, you will heal. Then, and only then, will you be capable of rebuilding your life. I'm living proof that it can be done. I was 47 when my beloved 49-yr-old husband died of a heart attack. Having experienced a happy marriage for 27 years, I knew what I was missing when it was gone. About a year later, I began my search to find another man with whom I could happily spend the remainder of my life. It took me 8 lonely years – 5 of them fervently devoted to my goal. Eventually, I found him.

I'm now remarried to a man who shares my love of classical music, laughter, people, beauty, literature and orderliness; a man with whom I've spent the past 16 years of my life. He has been my rock through good times and bad. Why he's still here is sometimes a mystery to me. It's hard to imagine the challenge it must be to live with a woman who develops new symptoms nearly every week. My illness has kept us from participating in many events he would have greatly enjoyed. Yet, he has cared more for my health than for his own pleasure. I feel so blessed to have found him, and I firmly believe we'll be together "until one lays the other in the arms of God". (That quote is from a country song I heard on the radio and never forgot. I wish I could remember the title.)

Some women are perfectly content to live alone or with a roommate, finding their happiness in their families and/or in their women friends. Others, like me, are happier with a male companion. Whatever your preference, my wish for each of you is to discover what makes you happy and to do whatever it takes to create it for yourself.

Whatever your choice, don't let FM get in your way. Keep reminding yourself that you have plenty to offer in any relationship, even though there will be days when you may have doubts about that. Those are the days when you must show as much compassion for yourself as you show to others. On your very worst day, you can still offer a welcoming smile and an empathetic ear. Those two things can be enough to make someone eager to come home to you.

Discussion Questions:

> *Have you suffered a loss and how did it affect your FM symptoms?*
> *What advice would you have for someone in a similar situation?*
> *What steps have been effective for you in overcoming grief?*

Chapter 36

The Beginning of the End
(Of life as I knew it)

Bolstered by the support of a wonderful group of women friends, I eased into life as a widow. I did a lot of soul searching in those days. I had worked hard to rise to my career as a financial analyst in an aerospace company from my humble beginning there as a secretary. I had completed my degree in the evening and attended all the training sessions the company offered. Many executive staff members sought my knowledge and expertise. But I never felt the satisfaction from my work that other people seemed to be feeling. Something was missing. I found myself applying the 20-year test to nearly everything I did. "In 20 years, who will care if this report gets submitted on time?" Or "In 20 years, who will care that I gave up my weekend to develop this budget?"

With the help of a wonderful therapist, I discovered I had a very deeply repressed, life-long goal. That goal was to become a physician. Growing up at a time when the only socially acceptable careers for women were teachers, nurses or secretaries, I had buried that desire so deeply that I was a middle-aged widow saddled with fibromyalgia by the time it emerged.

Even though I was feeling better physically than I had felt in years, I had to admit this goal wasn't doable for me. My symptoms could recur at any time. That had been the pattern for my entire life. So my goal remained a secret. I did go back to school again, but it was for a Master's program in Health Services Management.

My current employer subsequently offered me a temporary assignment at a satellite location some 50 miles away from my home. I hesitated at first, mostly because of the snowy winter weather. But the job site happened to be in my hometown where my recently widowed father still lived. I could stay with him during the week if I needed to, and it was a step up in my career. It sounded tailor made for me; I felt that I SHOULD take it. (There's that word again!)

I knew how lonely my father was. I could feel his pain. We were both struggling to adjust to losing a spouse and to living alone. Not having a job to go to made life even more lonely for him than it was for me. His days were filled with nothing but mourning. Living 50 miles away, I felt severe guilt for seeing him so seldom. Being there more often would mean that I could offer companionship, be sure that he ate balanced meals, and feel less regretful when I said "goodbye." It all sounded so good, but it was then that my life began to unravel.

The 50-mile commute was a nightmare - even though it averaged only two or three days a week. On those days, it meant a 10-hour rather than an 8-hour workday. I was far too tired to exercise when I got home. The effects were even worse the next day.

The pain and fatigue that had lain dormant for so long returned at that time with a vengeance. Concurrently, my cognitive difficulties began in earnest.

I just couldn't concentrate. I was learning a new job, trying to impress my new bosses, but it was taking me longer and longer to do less and less. Exhaustion was so constant and so severe that my eyes were blurry much of the time. Staying awake for dinner was a major accomplishment. The people who hired me must have regretted their choice. I just wanted my former life back.

By the time my temporary assignment was over, I was feeling really bad physically. I had the worst pain, the worst fatigue, and the worst IBS I'd ever experienced. However, I felt relieved to be back home, and I was confident that my health would improve once I resumed my routine and got back into the swimming pool. Wrong! The worst was yet to come.

In my absence, a new facility had been constructed specifically for the Top Secret government program to which I'd been assigned. A brand new office with all the latest computer equipment was constructed just for me. I should have been elated, but I was terrified instead. Why?

The new facility was built on the first floor of a 1940s-era factory at the far end of a facility the size of a football field. My office there was for use only when I was working on that Top Secret program. For all my other work (about a third of my day), my office was located in the extreme front of the building and on the second floor. There were no elevators in the building. Sounds bad, right? There's more.

The closest ladies' room to my newly-built Top Secret office was in the very center of the factory floor and up two very long flights of stairs. Stair climbing had been problematic for me for as long as I could remember - even when I was exercising regularly and feeling well. In my present condition, I feared my knees would buckle before I got to the top. Clearly, this situation was unworkable for someone with muscle fatigue and IBS.

At this point I had yet to tell anyone at work about my health issues. I had been conditioned by previous bosses to keep my personal problems to myself. So now I was really in a pickle. After only 6 months, I had to tell my new superiors that all the time and money they'd invested in my training had been a waste. I couldn't do my new job because of my health limitations and because there was no elevator. Talk about stress!

Fortunately, I had a friend in the company's medical office who told me about the Americans with Disabilities Act (ADA). The Act says that an employer must make a "reasonable accommodation" for a disabled employee. She assured me that some action would be taken as soon as she filed her report.

In the meantime, I wore super-strength sanitary pads to work in case I couldn't struggle up all those stairs in time. My pain was so bad, and my legs were so weak that I was usually in tears by the time I reached the top. Most days I went home early - as soon as I realized my legs wouldn't carry me up the stairs any more.

The "reasonable accommodation" the company made was to buy me an electric scooter so I could ride rather than walk to the closest first floor ladies room in the extreme front of the building all the way from my office in the extreme back of the building. Their logic was that this way I wouldn't need to climb stairs to get to a bathroom. Meanwhile, they would look for a new job assignment for me on the first floor.

My heart sank when I heard what their "accommodation" was. Remember, the distance to the foot of the stairs to the ladies room was the length of a football field, and those scooters don't go more than 5 miles an hour! Whoever came up with this idea surely never heard of IBS, especially IBS-D.

I knew it couldn't possibly work. I spent most of the next several months riding back and forth from my two offices. The remainder of the time I spent riding to and from the ladies room. It was ridiculous, and it was embarrassing. I endured pitying looks from my fellow employees. Almost daily I found myself skirting questions about why I was getting this special treatment.

There is a lesson to be learned here, however. It is that the ADA does work. If you need an accommodation in order to do your job, your employer must provide one (if the company employs 15 or more people). If climbing stairs where you work is difficult for you and is needlessly tiring you before the end of the day, talk to your supervisor about the Act. There may be workarounds that you never considered. Perhaps you could use a freight elevator (if there is one) or your tasks could be shared with another person who has no difficulty with stairs. You won't know if you don't ask.

Eventually I was reassigned to an office on the first floor of another building with a restroom just next door. My new bosses were great, allowing me to flex or reduce my hours as needed in order to attend doctor's appointments, physical therapy and swim. But, no matter how creatively I juggled my work schedule over the next few years, exercising and working on the same day proved to be just too exhausting for me. Working fewer hours didn't help either. That left me trying to accomplish the full-time tasks of a responsible job by working part-time hours. It was hugely stressful. It increased rather than decreased the severity of my symptoms.

I knew my working days were numbered, but I didn't want to admit it. Panic set in. As horrible as my life was, the alternative was even more frightening. But, eventually, the inevitable happened. After my second emergency hospitalization in two years, I finally accepted my reality and filed for long-term disability.

Discussion Questions:

> *If you're still working, what challenges do you face?*
> *Have you utilized the ADA? How successfully?*
> *If you're on disability, how difficult was that decision for you to make?*

Chapter 37

The End of the Beginning

I never did become a physician. More than 19 years after claiming disability my cognitive functioning and my level of fatigue haven't improved all that much. Once I'd adjusted to being unemployed for a while, I tried to take a class on the Internet. Even that was a huge challenge for me. My deficient short-term memory was difficult to overcome.

For a time, I sank into a deep depression. I felt like my life had been a sham. I did all the things society expected a dutiful girl to do: got married, had a child, stayed at home or worked at mindless jobs that conformed to my child's school schedule, chaired the PTA, and cared for my home and my family. Eventually, I worked full-time and even earned a graduate degree. I did all the SHOULDS, but I never lived for me.

No one ever asked me what I wanted to do with my life. Had they done so, I couldn't have answered the question. As a child I had no female role models who did anything other than stay home and raise a family. My one childless aunt lived several states away. She had an exciting life with her military husband. They travelled the world and seemed very happy to me. I thought her lifestyle was idyllic, but because I saw her so seldom, her existence didn't represent reality to me.

As a young woman with a family of my own but no immediate family close by, I honestly didn't believe there were options. I never considered going back to school at that time. I took my mothering obligations too seriously. Leaving a child with a babysitter (even if we could have afforded one) while I went back to school and my husband went to work would have been unthinkable – even if I'd been motivated to do it.

After graduating from high school, my practical father said I could go to a 2-year college, so that's what I did. His belief was that a woman didn't really need an education or the ability to support herself. That was the reason for having a husband. Earning an Associates Degree was just insurance in case a tragedy occurred and she needed to be employed. It was the way the world worked in the 60's, at least in my view (which was my family's view) of the world.

Thankfully, I'd later gone to work for a large corporation which offered college tuition for its employees, and I'd taken advantage of it. While my son was in high school, I went back to school at night, earning a bachelor's and later a master's degree. My efforts were recognized by my employer, and my career was launched.

Fast forward to filing for disability. There I was, totally alone - having lost my husband, my career, my friends and even my dreams. My only child was working in New York City, some five hours away, well on his way to a successful legal career. I was very proud of his accomplishments, but I missed him dearly. My only sibling lived several hours away and spent most of her life travelling the world with her husband for whom it was a job requirement.

To finally have recognized my life's ambition to be a physician and then have to admit that it was an impossible goal was yet another painful loss. No 50-

year-old medical student with severe symptoms of fibromyalgia could survive the life of an intern. It felt a bit like losing myself - after I'd just been discovered.

So, for the first time in my life, I had to look into the mirror and ask, "Who is this woman, this former striving financial analyst, would-be physician, ardent writer and devoted mother?

I am a survivor who made a decision to improve her life and moved clear across the country to do so. I have finally made peace with my physical and mental limitations, and I'm determined to do something positive with my life.

Writing this book is one way I've chosen to do it. The countless hours I've struggled to put this book together has resulted in one of my greatest achievements. If I've motivated even one person to take a trip or to plant a garden; if I've assisted a person in filing for disability, if I've allayed one person's fear of narcotic addiction, inspired someone to watch a sunset, do laughter yoga or learn to meditate, then I will have achieved my goal.

I will have finally passed the "20-year-test." In 20 years, who will care that I persevered thru the pain, fatigue and cognitive challenges of fibromyalgia in order to write this book? That one person whose life I touched will care! And I will consider my life a success.

Epilogue

So, what's next? I've pondered this question since I saw this book coming to a conclusion. I know now that I was born to write. It totally absorbs my attention. Hours slip magically by without my realizing it whenever I sit at my keyboard. Writing is responsible for getting me through painful feelings and difficult times. But, even more, I'd like to think that my writing serves a helpful purpose for others.

Now I'm ready to try something new. From talking to other fibromyalgia sufferers I've learned that many of them would rather listen to a recorded book than to read one. After considering that fact and realizing my voice (narrating and singing) has always been one of my best assets, I've decided to narrate this book to create an audio version.

There will be a learning curve to efficiently operate the required equipment and to navigate recording software I've never seen before. But I'm hoping it will be a successful effort that will lead to a new opportunity. Narrating books for other authors is a future goal of mine. I intend to give it my best effort. If I'm successful, then it was meant to be. If I'm not, at least I've learned some new skills and faced a new challenge successfully.

Regardless of what else I do, I'd like to continue to help newly-diagnosed FM sufferers. I'd like to learn more about the person inside me I've never known and to add a great deal of laughter and adventure to my life. None of us knows which of our days will be our last. My foremost intention is to spend my last days smiling. My wish is that you will, too.

Appendix A
Recommended Reading List

About Fibromyalgia

The Arthritis Foundation's Guide to Alternative Therapies, Judith Horstman

The Arthritis Helpbook, Kate Lorig, R.N. and James F. Fries, M.D.

Breaking Thru the Fibro Fog, Kevin P. White, MD, PhD

Fibromyalgia & Chronic Myofascial Pain Syndrome, Devin Starlanyl, M.D. and Mary Ellen Copeland

The Divided Mind, John Sarno, M.D.

The Fibromyalgia Dental Handbook, Flora Parsa Stay, D.D.S.

From Fatigued to Fantastic, Jacob Teitelbaum, M.D.

Your Personal Guide to Living Well with Fibromyalgia, The Arthritis Foundation

Natural Choices for Fibromyalgia, Jane Oelke, N.D., Ph.D.

Arthritis Today Magazine

www.co-cure.org

fibromyalgialatest.com

www.FibromalgiaNewsToday.com

About Feeling Better

Aromatherapy for Everyone, PJ Pierson and Mary Shipley

Feeling Good, The New Mood Therapy, David Burns, M.D.

Full Catastrophe Living, Jon Kabat-Zinn, Ph.D.

Getting to the Other Side of Grief, Susan Zonnebelt-Smeenge, R.N. Ed.D. and Robert DeVries, D.Min, Ph.D.

I Thought It Was Just Me, Brenee Brown

Loving What Is, Byron Katie

Managing Pain before it Manages You, Margaret A. Caudill, MD, Ph.D., MPH

Meditations for Women Who Do Too Much, Ann Schaef

Mind Over Medicine, Lissa Rankin, M.D.

Perfect Health, Deepak Chopra, M.D.

Reversing Chronic Pain, Maggie Phillips

Secrets to Self Healing, Dr. Maoshing Ni

Sleep Disorders, Dr. K. Roth

Spontaneous Healing, Andrew Weil, M.D.

Staying Well with Guided Imagery, Belleruth Naperstek

The Power of Breath: The Art of Breathing Well for Harmony, Happiness & Health, Swami Saradananda

The Power of Now, Eckhart Tolle

The Psychology of Achievement, Brian Tracy

You Can Heal Your Life, Louise Hay (book or kindle editions)

www.patientslikeme.com

About Eating Better

The Body Ecology Diet, Donna Gates

Grain Brain, David Perlmutter, M.D.

Gut Solutions, Watson & Smith

Power Nutrition for Your Chronic Illness, Kristine Napier, M.P.H., R.D.

Foods that Fight Pain, Dr. Neal Barnard

Healing with Whole Foods, Paul Pitchford

Wheat Belly Total Health, William Davis, M.D.

Appendix B
Daily FM Diary

Daily FM Diary

	1	2	3	4	5	6	7	8	9	10
RATE YOUR SLEEP										
# Hrs. _____										
# Interruptions _____										
# Naps yesterday _____	Good ○	○	○	○	ok ○	○	○	○	○	Poor ○
RATE YOUR SYMPTOMS										
PAIN	Tolerable ○	○	○	○	Achy ○	○	○	○	○	Awful ○
FATIGUE	Not bad ○	○	○	○	Tired ○	○	○	○	○	Exhausted ○
BOWEL FUNCTION	Constipated ○	○	○	○	Normal ○	○	○	○	○	Diarrhea ○
RATE YOUR STATE OF MIND										
ANXIETY	Calm ○	○	○	○	○	A little tense ○	○	○	○	Stressed ○
DEPRESSION	Happy ○	○	○	○	○	A little blue ○	○	○	○	Hopeless ○
CONFUSION	Clear Mind ○	○	○	○	Fuzzy ○	○	○	○	○	Fibrofog ○
RATE YOUR FUNCTIONAL ABILITY										
WALKING	Good to go ○	○	○	○	○	1 block only ○	○	○	Can barely stand ○	○
READING	ok ○	○	○	○	○	Hard to focus ○	○	○	○	Total blur ○
RATE CONTRIBUTING FACTORS										
TEMPERATURE	Cold ○	○	○	○	Mild ○	○	○	○	○	Hot ○
HUMIDITY	Dry ○	○	○	○	Humid ○	○	○	○	○	Rain/Snow ○
SKY	Gloomy ○	○	○	○	Cloudy ○	○	○	○	○	Sunny ○
SMOG	Clear ○	○	○	○	Light Smog ○	○	○	○	○	High Alert ○
POLLEN COUNT	Low ○	○	○	○	Normal ○	○	○	○	○	High ○
SITUATIONAL STRESS	All is well ○	○	○	○	○	A Bit Tense ○	○	○	○	Total Chaos ○

Where does it hurt? Mark with "X"

DATE _____ a.m./p.m.

General Health (Circle One) Good Fair Poor

273

Appendix C
Physician's FM Disability Questionnaire

Patient: _____

Soc. Sec.#: _____

How long have you known this patient?_____

Frequency of contact

_____

Does your patient meet the ACR Criteria for FMS?

                    Yes   No

List Any other diagnosed impairments:

_____

Have your patient's impairments lasted or are they expected to last at least 12 months?

                    Yes   No

Clinical Findings, Lab/Test Results

_____

If your Patient has Pain, where is it located?

_____

Describe the frequency and severity of your patient's pain:

_____

Circle any factors that precipitate pain:

Weather	Fatigue	Repetitive Motion
Stress	Cold	Hormonal Changes
Humidity	Heat	Static Position
Allergies	Other: _____	

275

Is your patient a malingerer?   Yes   No

What side effects of patient's pain medications have implications for working? For example, drowsiness, diarrhea, stomach upset, dizziness, etc.

_____

What functional limitations would your patient have in a work situation?

_____

Does your patient need a job that allows shifting positions at will from standing, sitting, walking, etc.?
                                   Yes   No
Will your patient sometimes need to lie down at unpredictable intervals during a work shift?
                                   Yes   No
While standing/walking, must your patient use a cane or other assistive device?
                         Yes   No   Sometimes

On average, how often do you anticipate that your patient's impairments and/or treatments would cause the patient to be absent from work?
Never Less than once/mo.   More than 3 times/mo.

Describe any other limitations that would affect this patient's ability to work at a regular job on a sustained basis:

_____

_____

Signed:_____Date:_____

Print/Type Name:

_____Phone:_____

Address:_____

_____

Appendix D
Exercises for the Pool

Important Reminders

- Check with your doctor before beginning any exercise program.
- Stop if you feel any pain.
- Keep your arms in the water.
- Concentrate on stretching to increase your range of motion.
- Do not repeat any motion more than twice in a row.
- Quit before you feel tired.
- Do a different form of exercise tomorrow (i.e. walk).

Begin with a warm up — 5 minutes of water walking in chest-deep water. Walk several steps forward, and then back. Side step to the right, and then back. Side step to the left, and then back.

At the Side of the Pool (Shoulder-deep water)

1. Back against the side: Arms at shoulder height: Stretch arms out to the side. Then cross in front and hug yourself. Repeat.
2. Holding side with left hand: With weight on left leg, keeping right arm and leg straight, lift arm and leg forward, then swing back behind you, pendulum- style. Repeat. Turn and switch sides.
3. Back against the side: Lift right knee toward chest. Hold with right arm for 3 seconds. Release. Switch legs.
4. Hands against the sides: Arms straight. Feet 2 feet from wall. Bend elbows, bringing face toward wall. Straighten elbows. Repeat.
5. Back against the side: Cross legs, one at a time, in front of you, then out to the side. Repeat.
6. Repeat from "At the Side of the Pool #1."

In Deeper Water (Using a Tube or a Noodle)

1. Bicycle kick slowly for 2 minutes.
2. Criss-cross legs, first right over left, then left over right slowly. Repeat.
3. Scissor kick, right leg forward, left leg back. Reverse.
4. Legs hanging vertically, flex your feet up, then down. Toes out, then in. Heels out, then in. Repeat.
5. March in place for 3 minutes, raising your knees as high as possible.
6. Use your right big toe to draw a circle. Reverse the circle. Do the same with your left big toe. Repeat.
7. Use your right foot to draw a larger circle. Reverse. Do the same with your left. Repeat.
8. Repeat from "In Deeper Water #1."

In Waist High Water (Legs shoulder-width apart. Hips facing forward.)

1. Hands on hips: Rotate at the waist to right. Look at the wall behind you. Hold 5 seconds, and then come back to center. Then repeat on the left side. Repeat.
2. Hands on hips: Bend over to your right. Hold for 3 seconds. Straighten up slowly. Repeat on the left.
3. Hands on hips: Looking straight ahead. Lower right ear to shoulder. Hold 3 seconds, and then lift head. Lower left ear to shoulder. Hold 3 seconds. Repeat.
4. Hands at your sides: Slide your right hand down the side of your right leg, bending at the waist. Hold briefly. Straighten up slowly. Repeat on the left.
5. Repeat from "In Waist High Water #1."
6. **End with a Cool Down** (in chest-deep water)
7. Walk several steps forward, and then back. Sidestep to the right, then back. Sidestep to the left, then back. Repeat for 5 minutes.

Index

About the Author

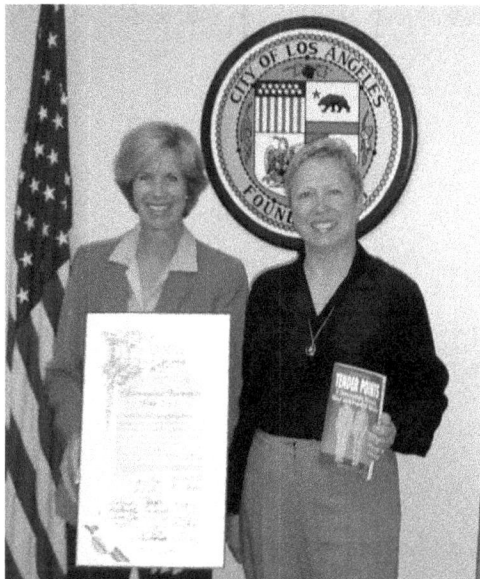

Christine Danella Lynch (seen here with then CA Congressperson, and currently L.A. County Supervisor, Janice Hahn) declaring May 12 to be National Fibromyalgia Day in Los Angeles, California. Diagnosed with fibromyalgia in 1990, Lynch has experienced its symptoms since childhood. Severe physical and cognitive difficulties ended her career as a corporate financial analyst and prompted her claim for disability. Lynch was trained as an FM support group leader by the Arthritis Foundation and has participated in FM support groups on both the east and west coasts. She is a National Fibromyalgia Association Leader Against Pain and has lobbied for increased funding for research and support for fibromyalgia patients in Sacramento. She currently writes a weekly column for the online publication, "Fibromyalgia News Today". Her column is entitled Tender Points.